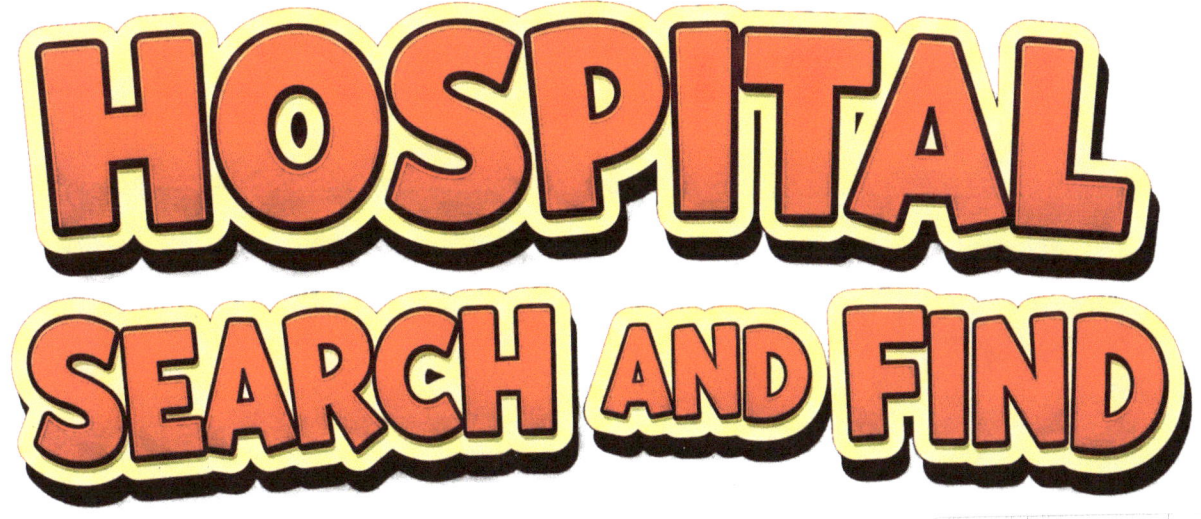

This book belongs to:

By Dr. Fei Zheng-Ward   Illustrated by Emily Skinner

Copyright © 2025 Fei Zheng-Ward

All rights reserved. Published by Fei Zheng-Ward, an imprint of FZWbooks. No part of this book may be copied, reproduced, recorded, transmitted, or stored by any means or in any form, electronic or mechanical, without obtaining prior written permission from the copyright owner.

<u>Disclaimer</u>: Please note that the illustrations are not drawn to scale.

This book is for informational, educational, personal growth, and entertainment purposes and should not be used as a substitute for medical advice.

The author and the publisher are not responsible, either directly or indirectly, for any damages, monetary losses, or reparations due to information in this book. By reading this book, the readers agree not to hold the author and the publisher responsible for any losses as a result of any errors, inaccuracies, or omissions in this book.

Identifier: ISBN 979-8-89318-084-8 (paperback)
            ISBN 979-8-89318-092-3 (hardcover)

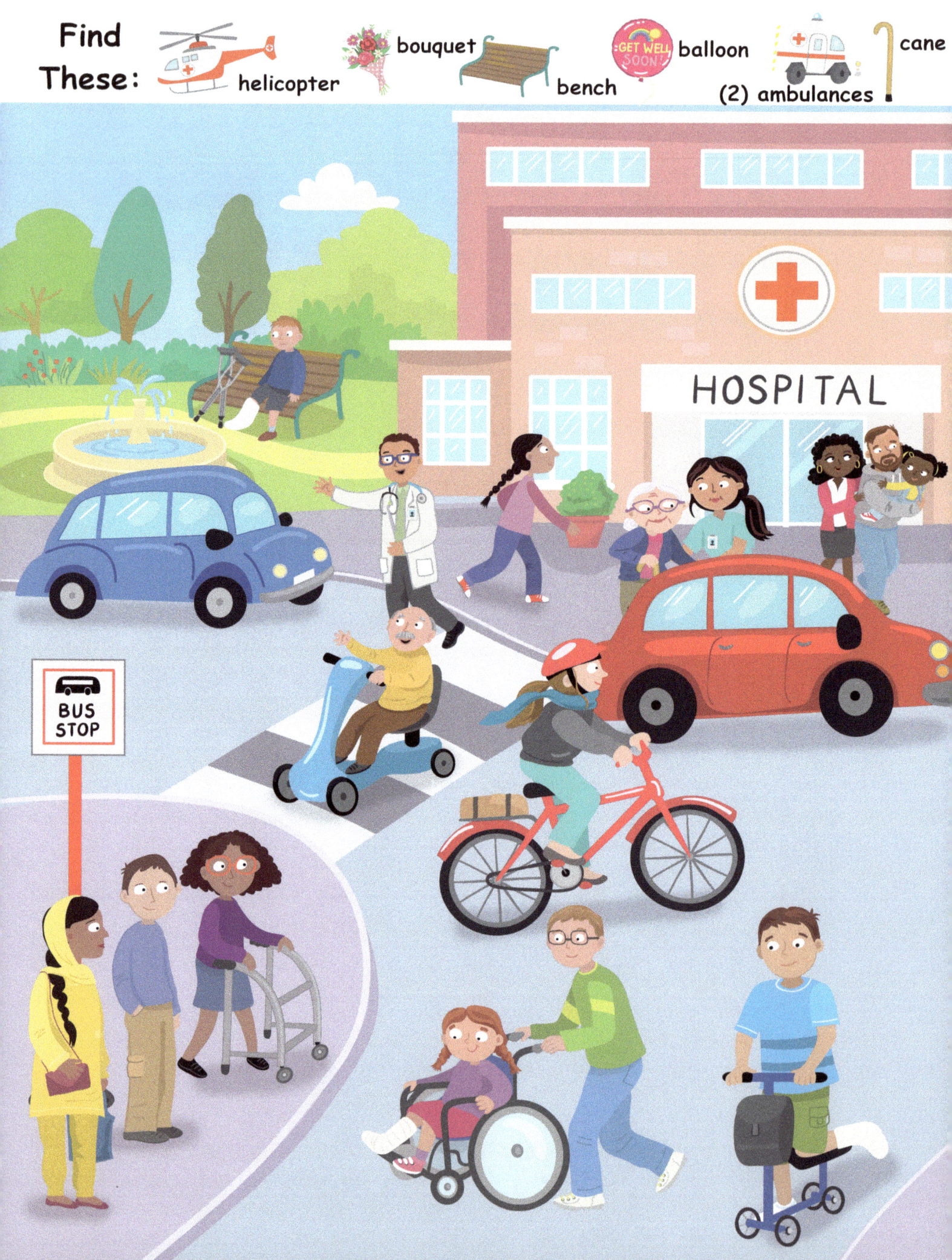

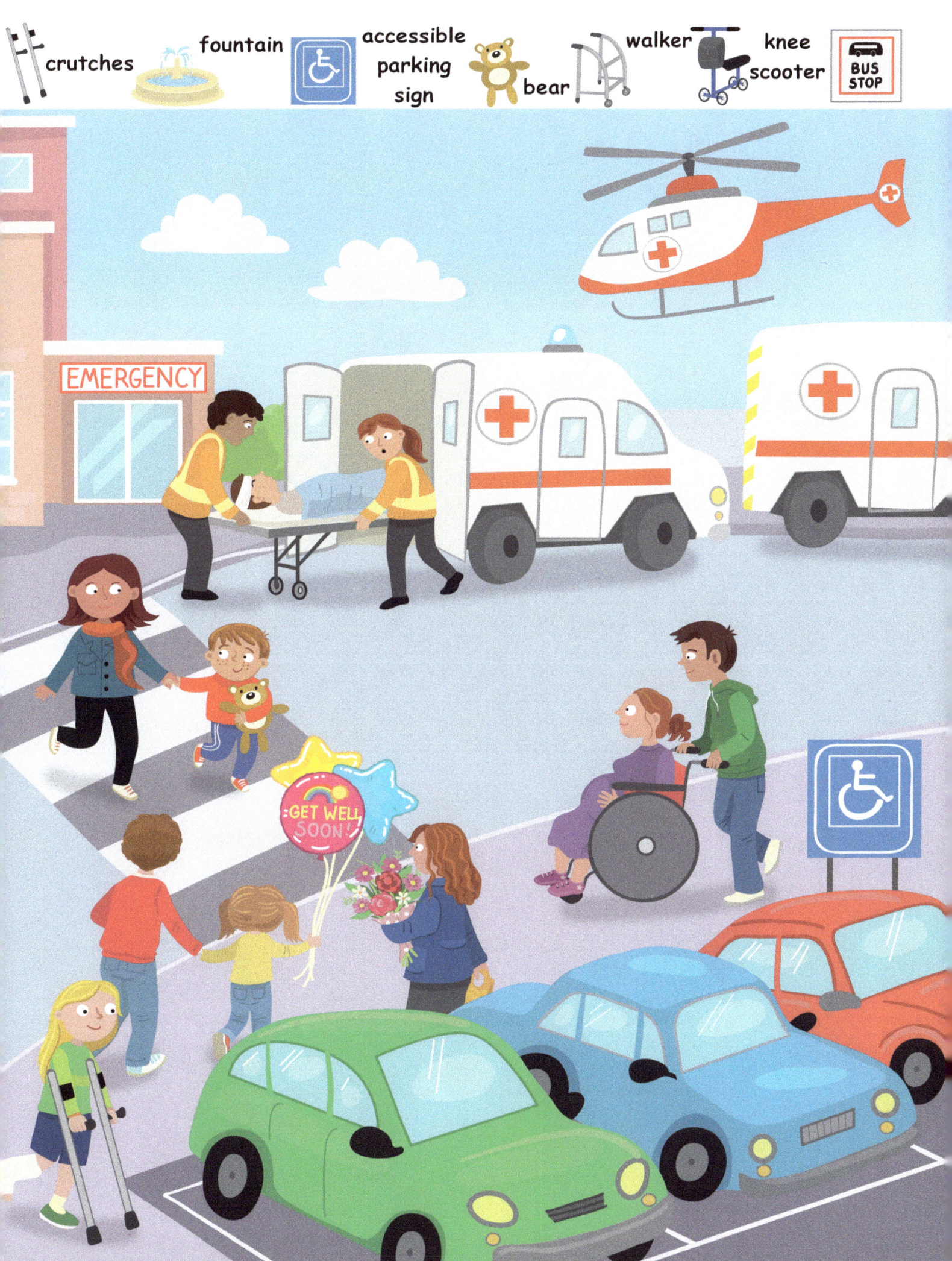

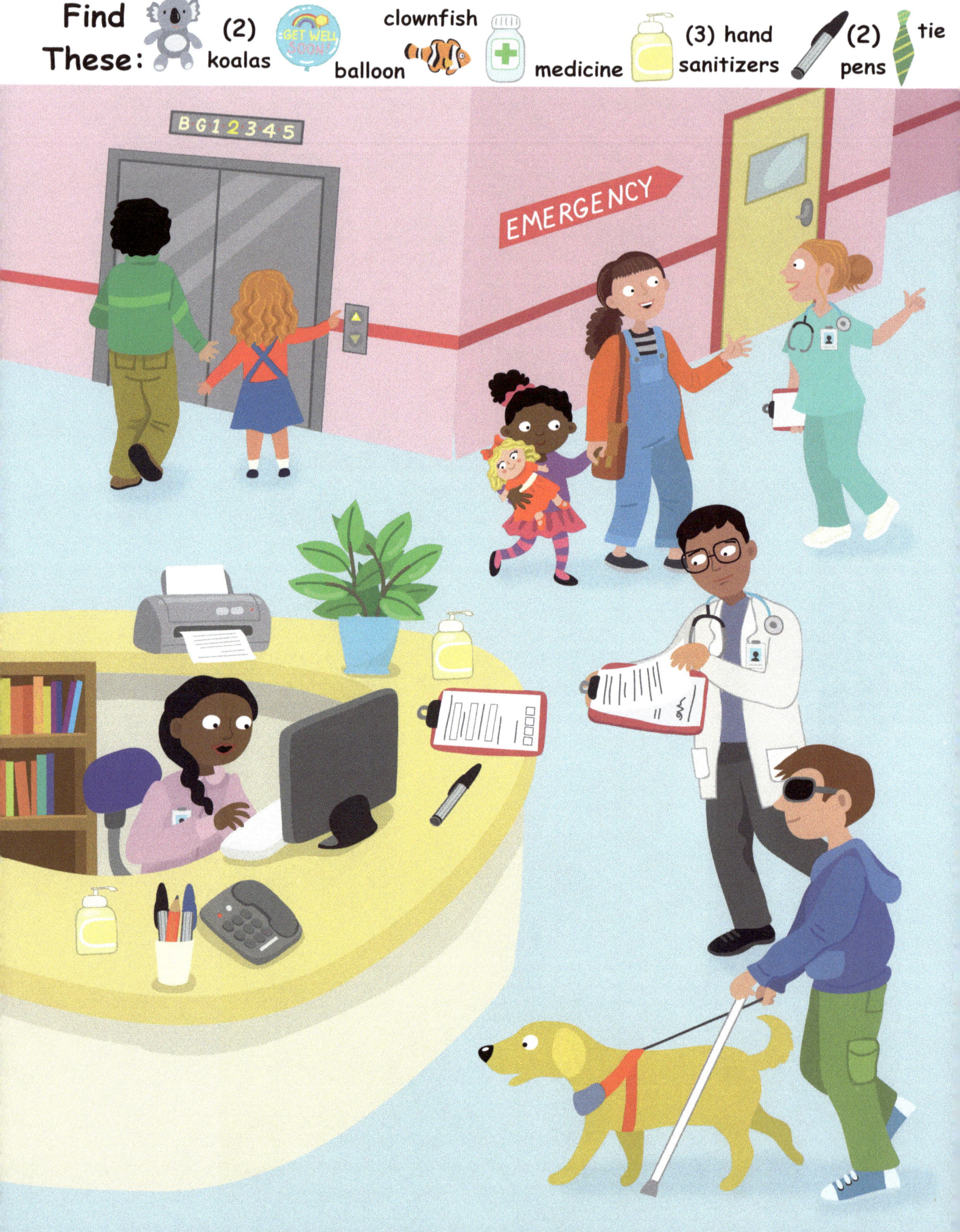

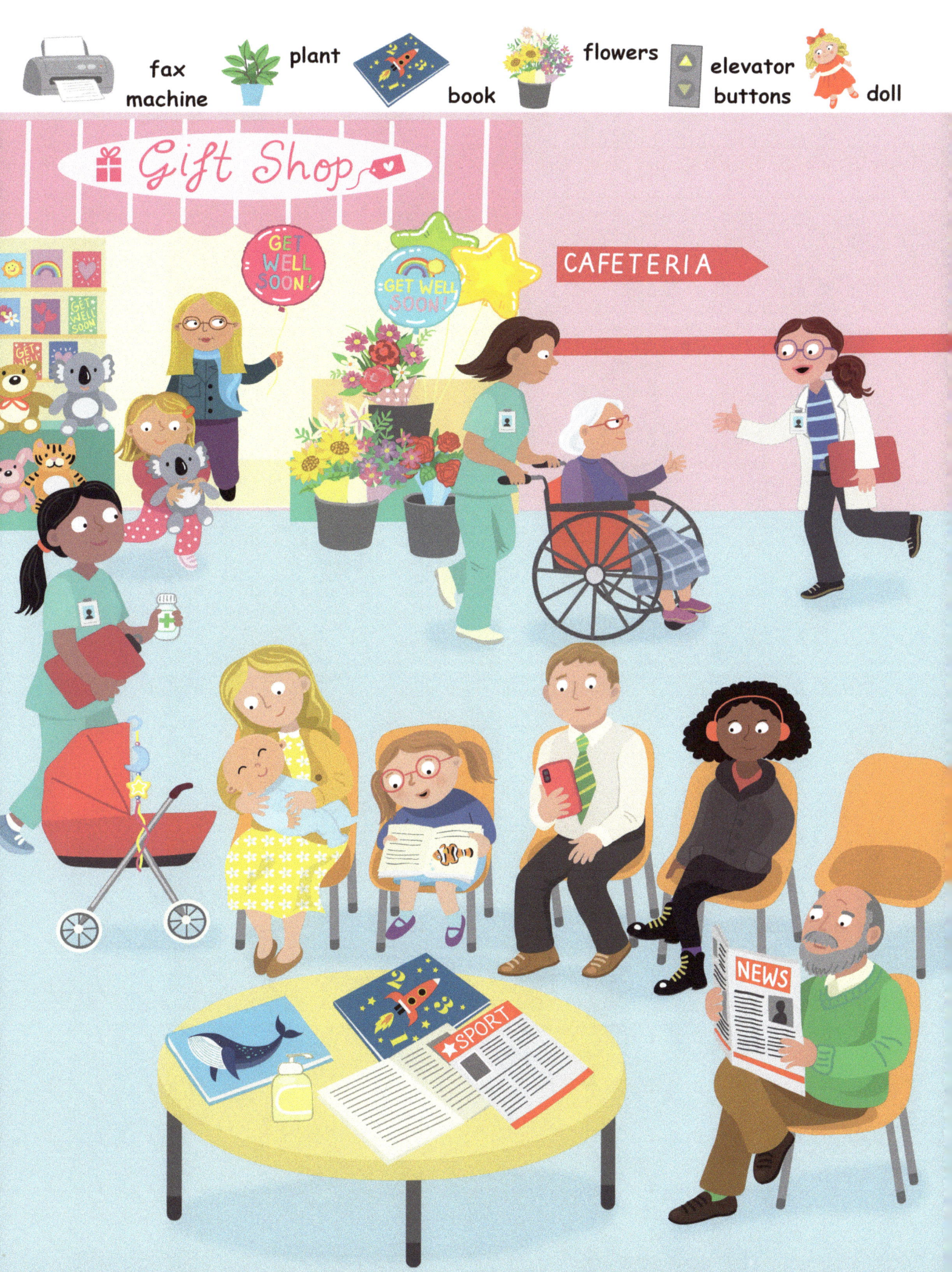

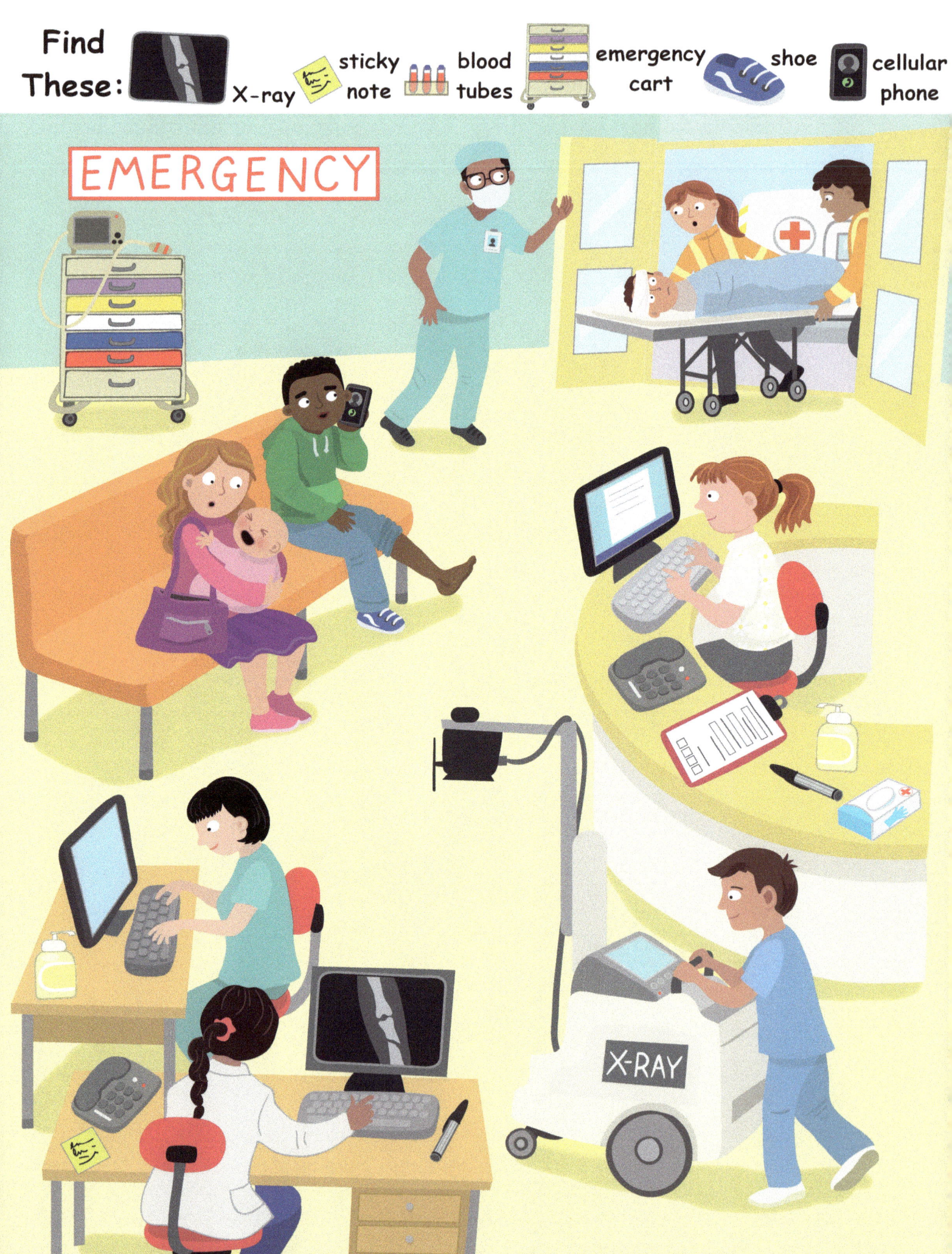

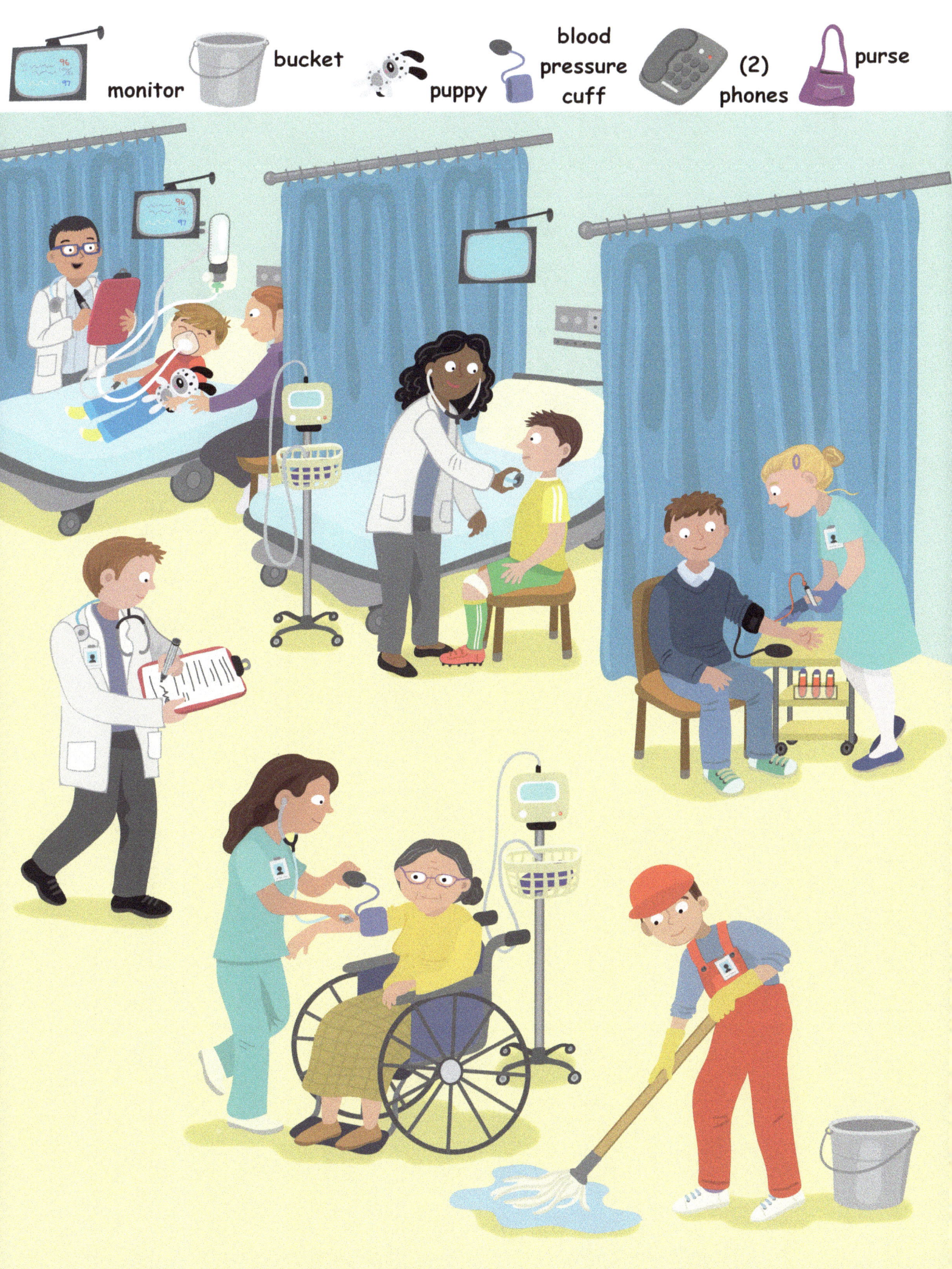

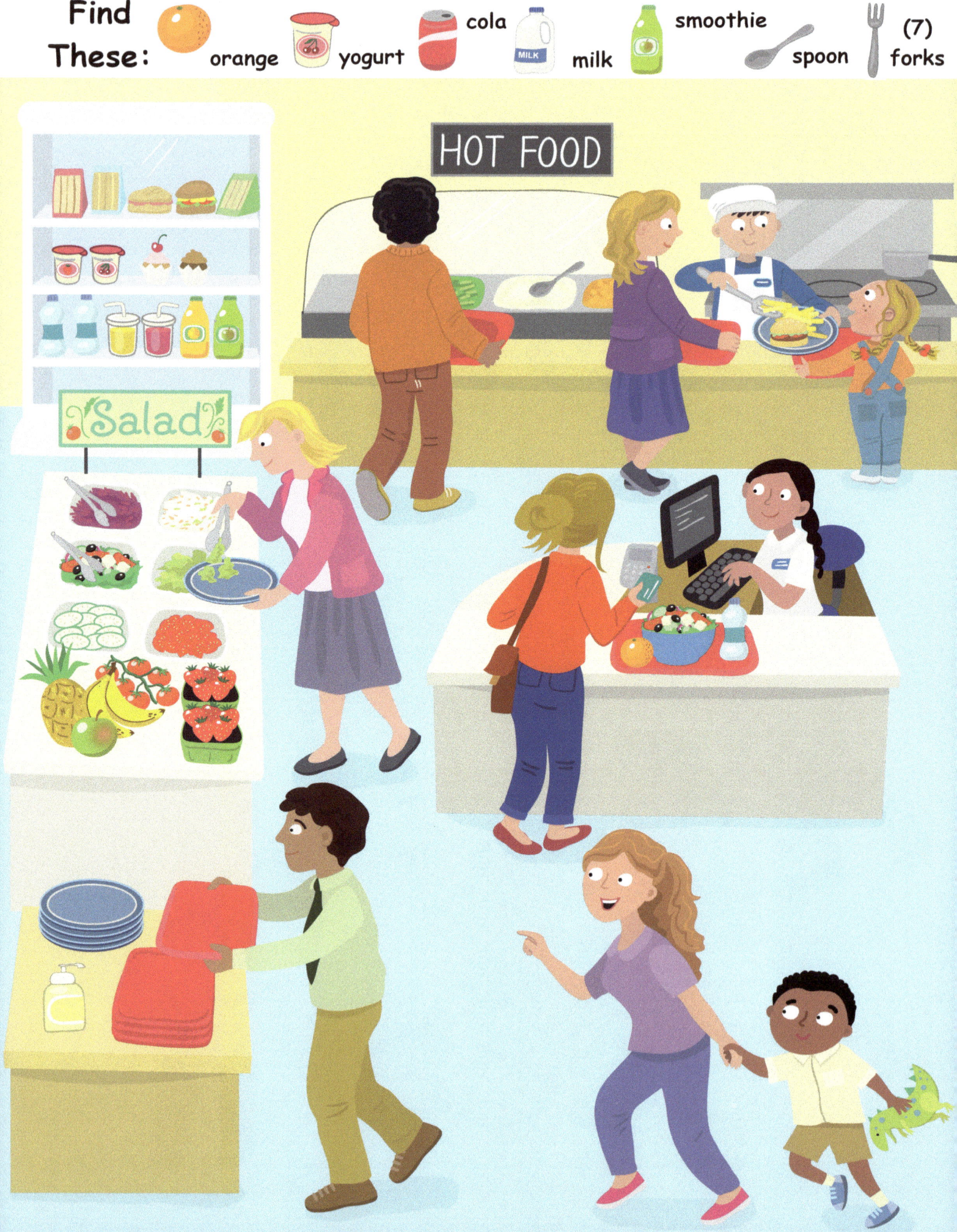

(8) waters | hot dog | spaghetti with sauce | (2) hamburgers | dino

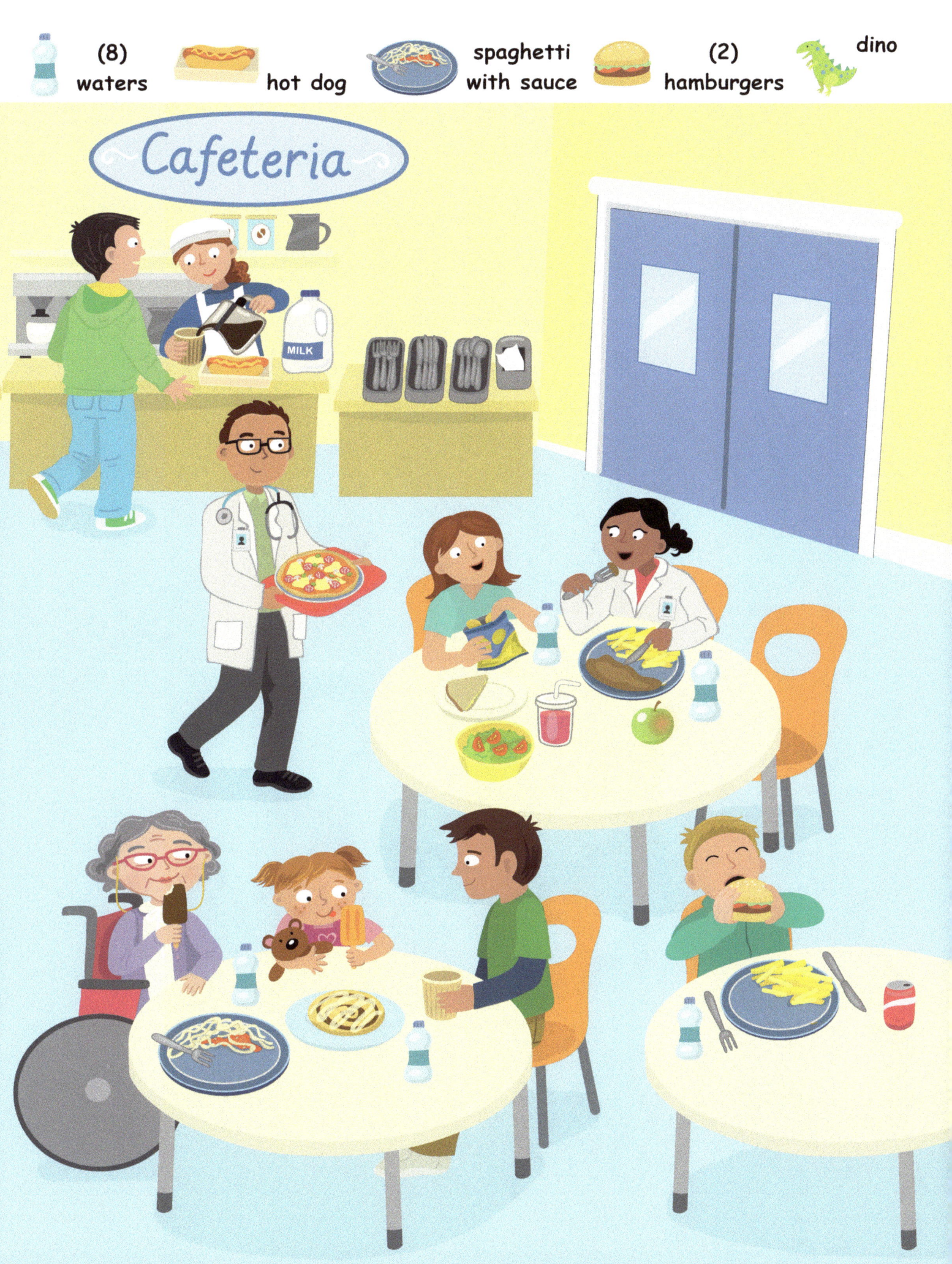

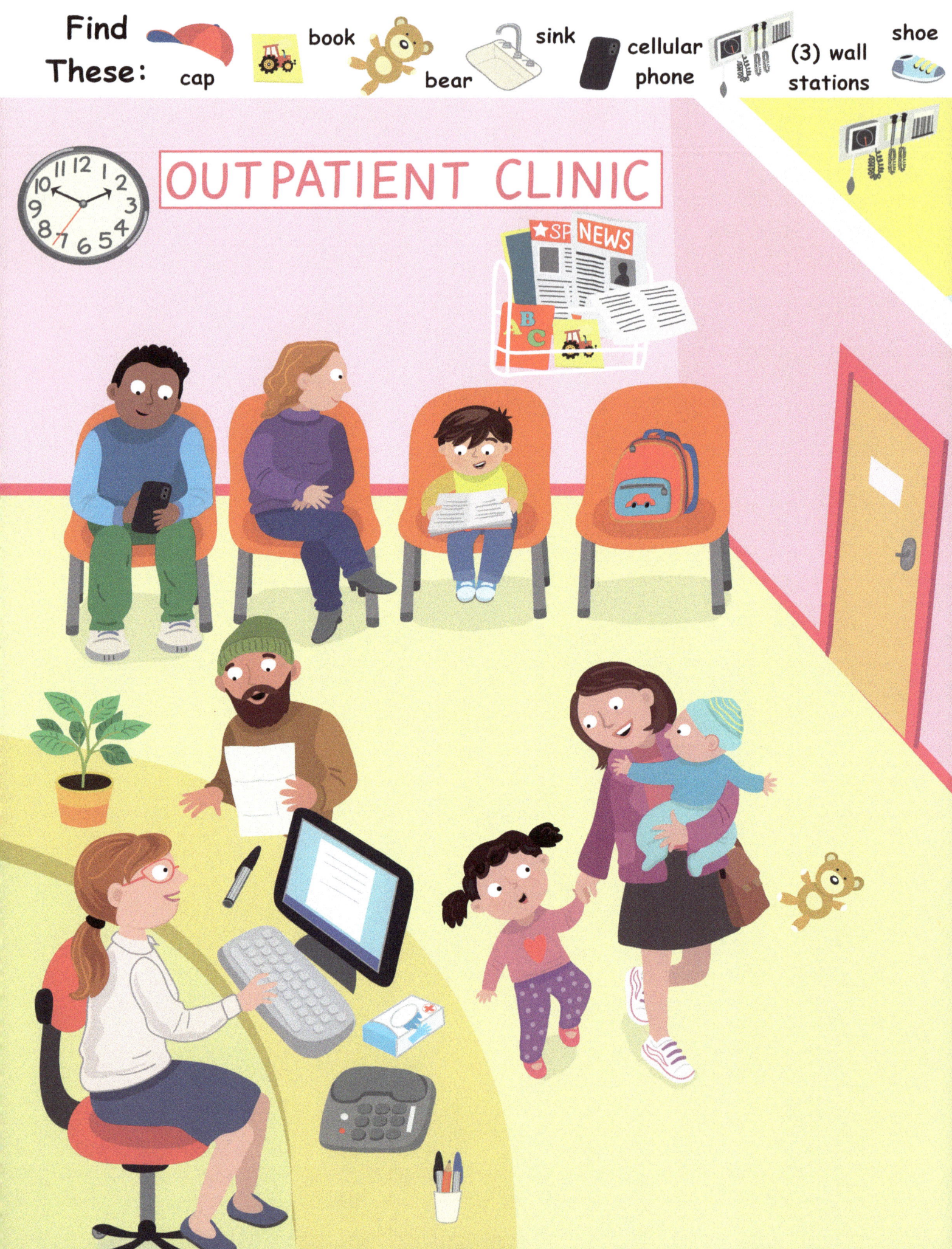

newspaper and book rack | (2) linen bins | backpack | (4) boxes of gloves | beanie

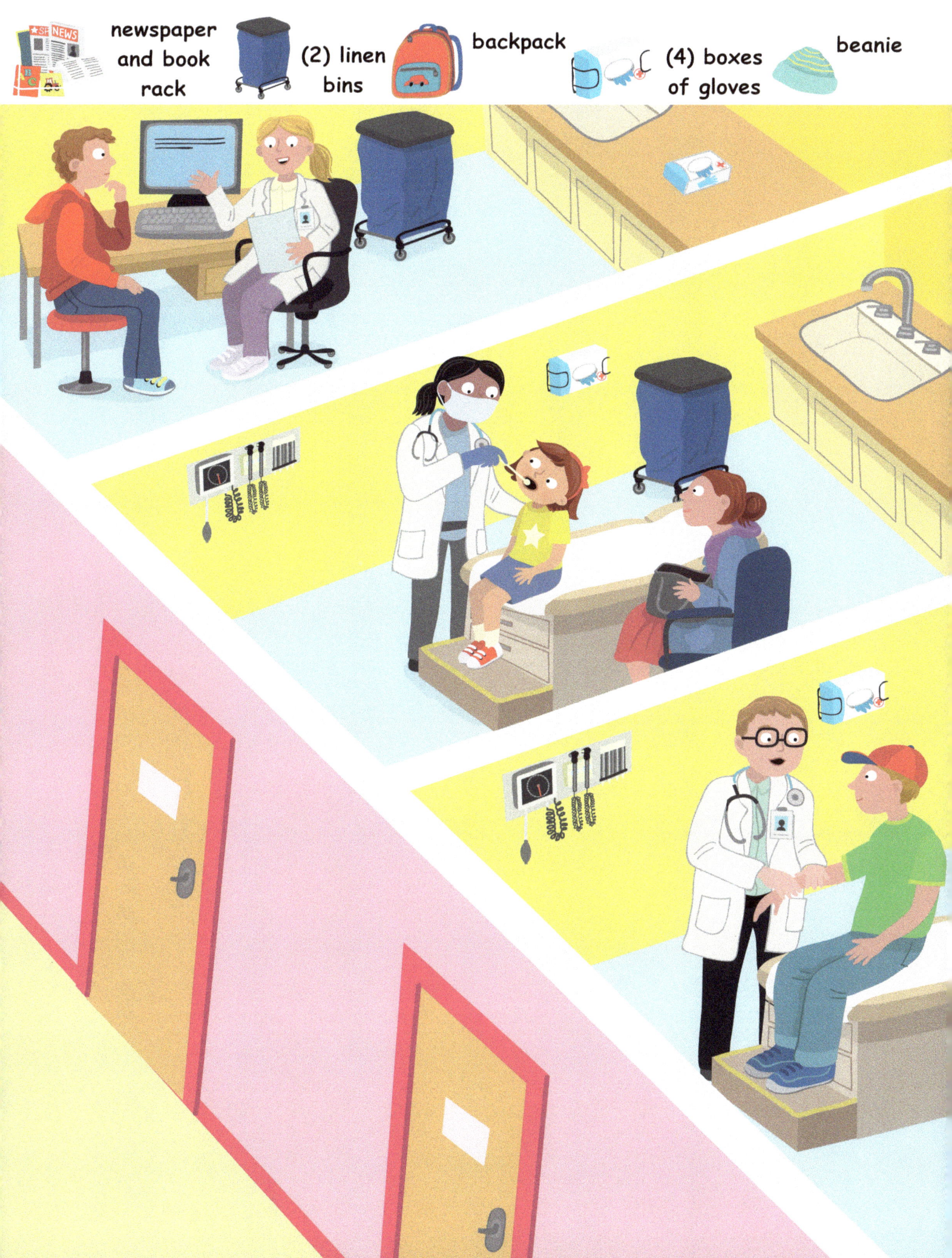

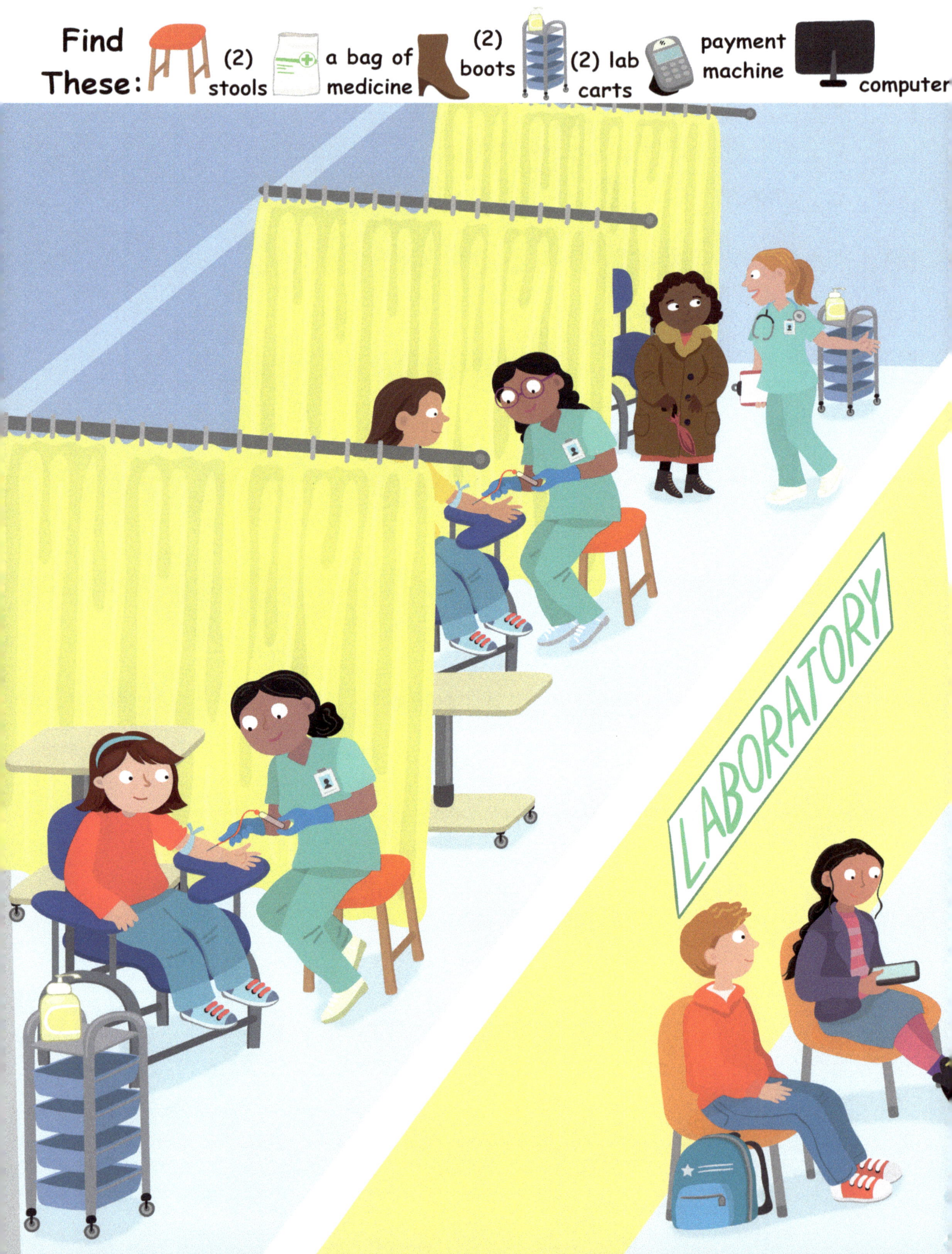

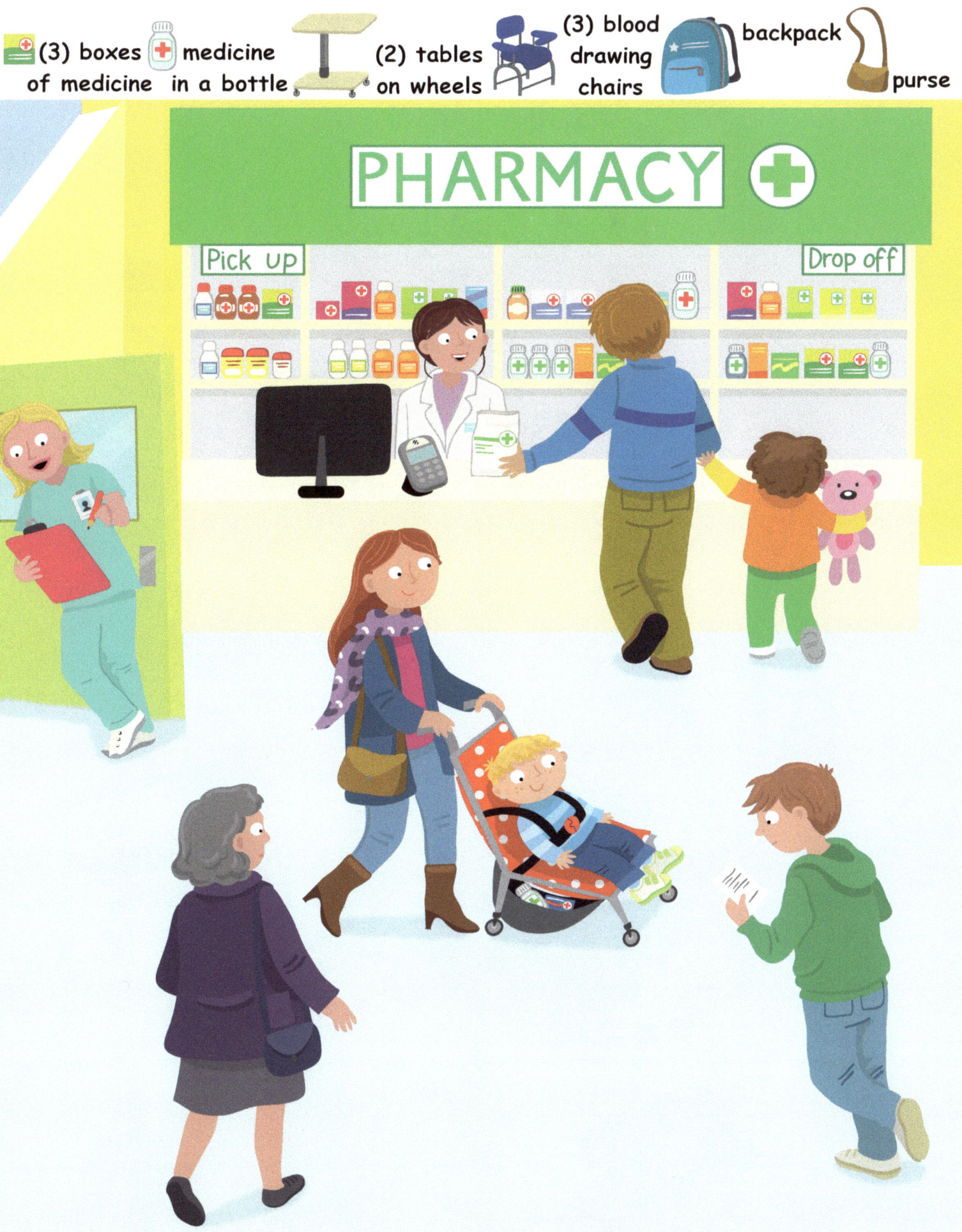

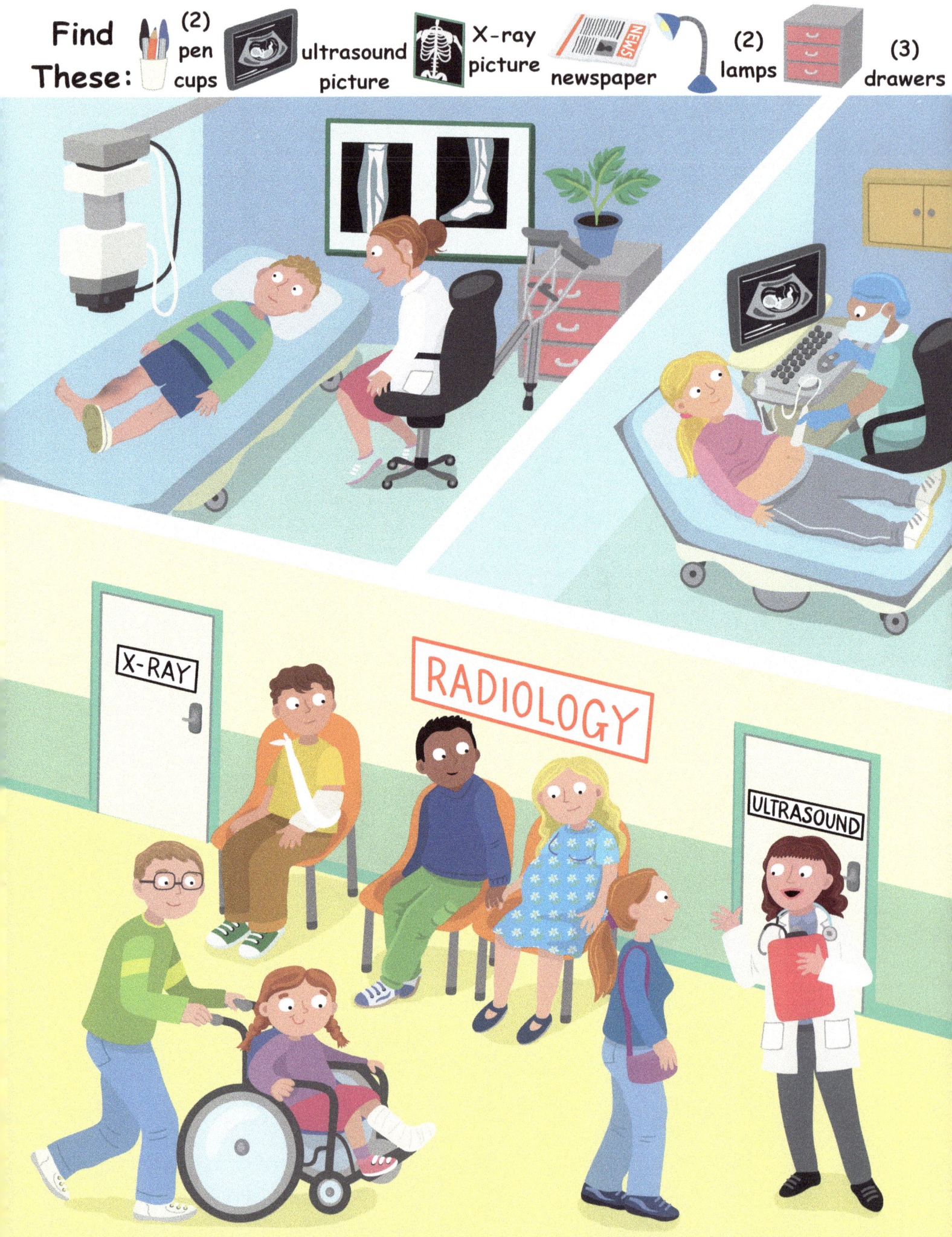

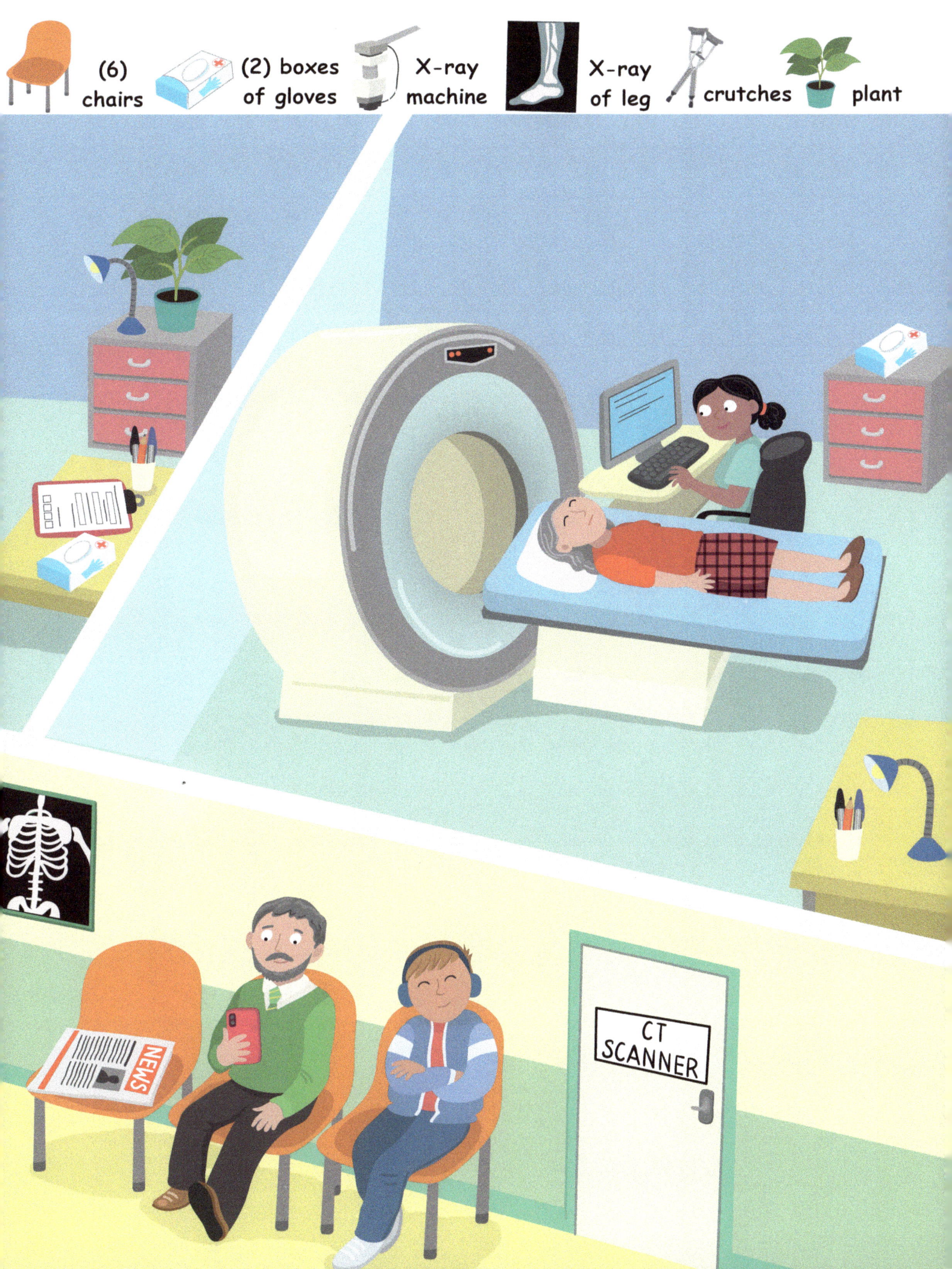

Find These: (3) vital signs monitors, (2) boxes of gloves, waste basket, doctor's notes, laptop, scissors

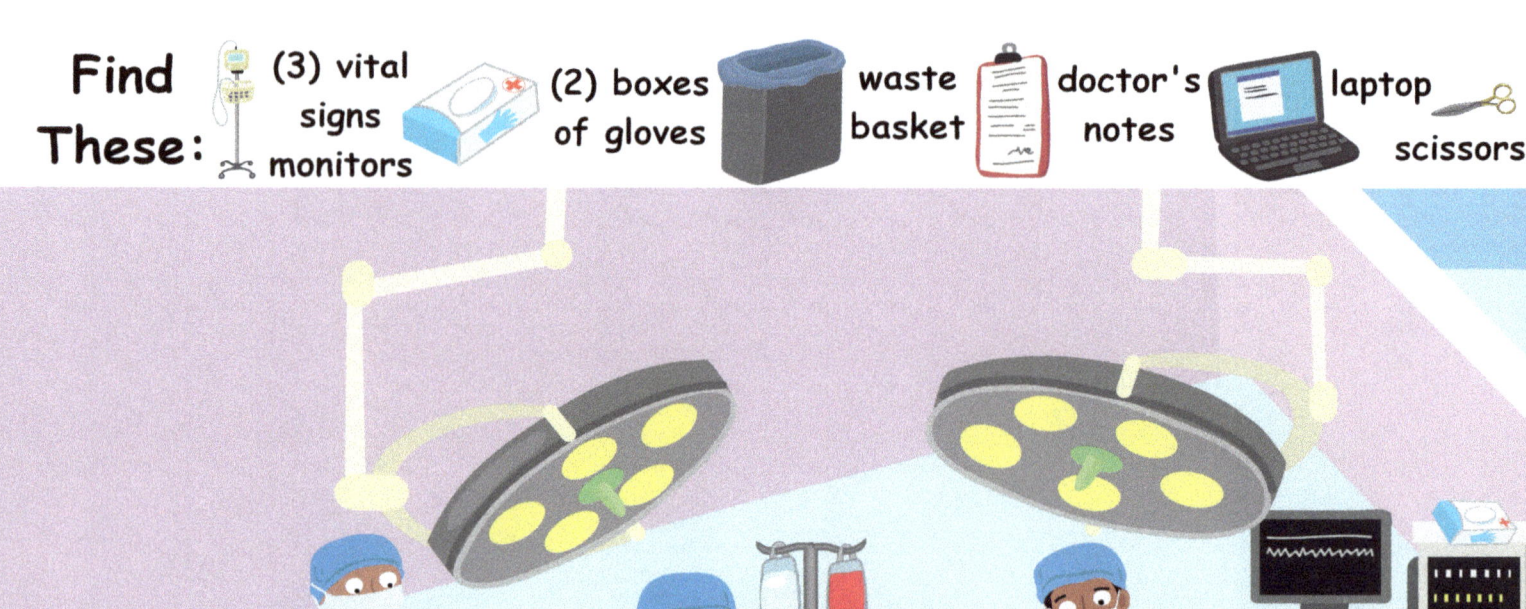

OPERATING ROOM

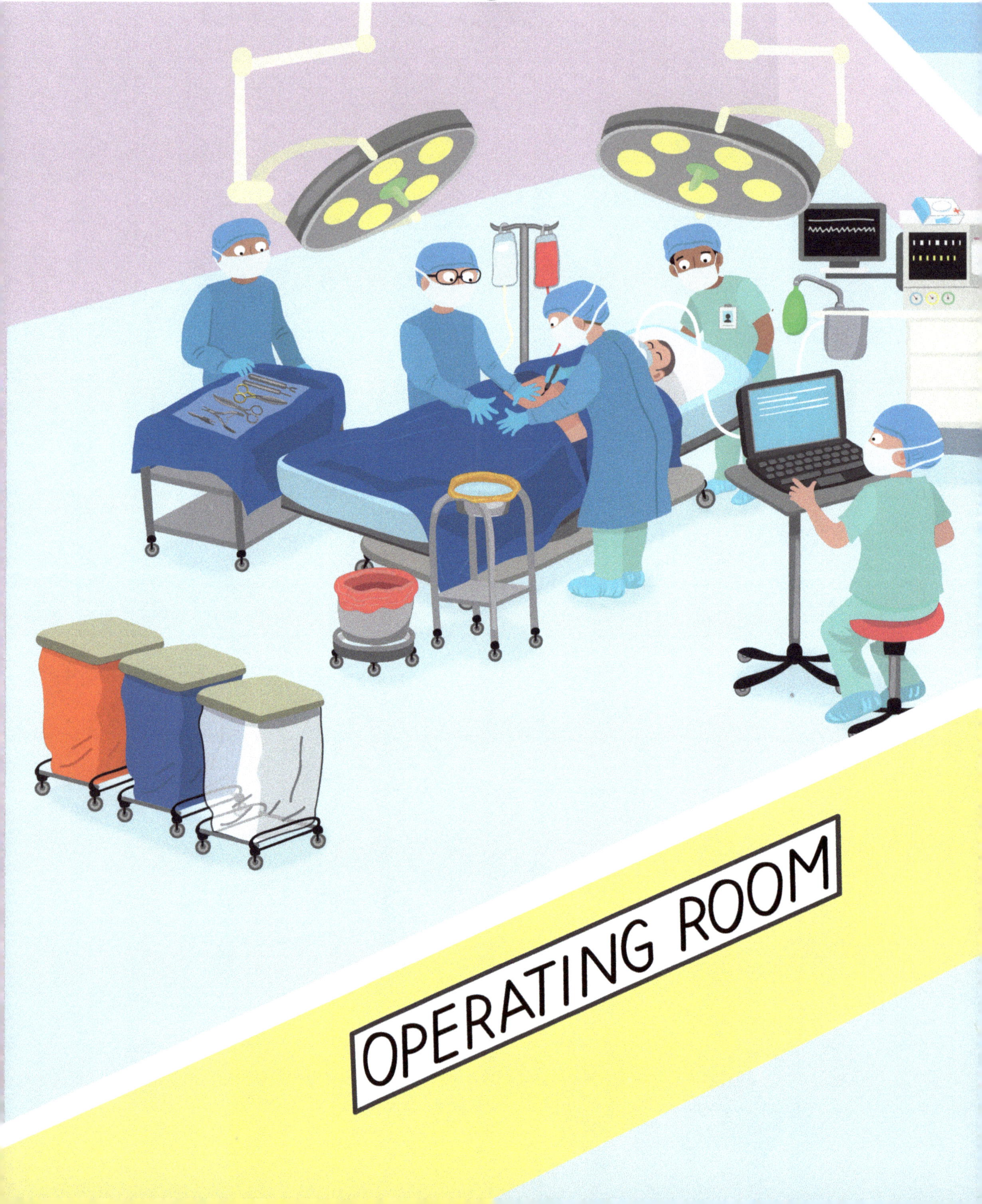

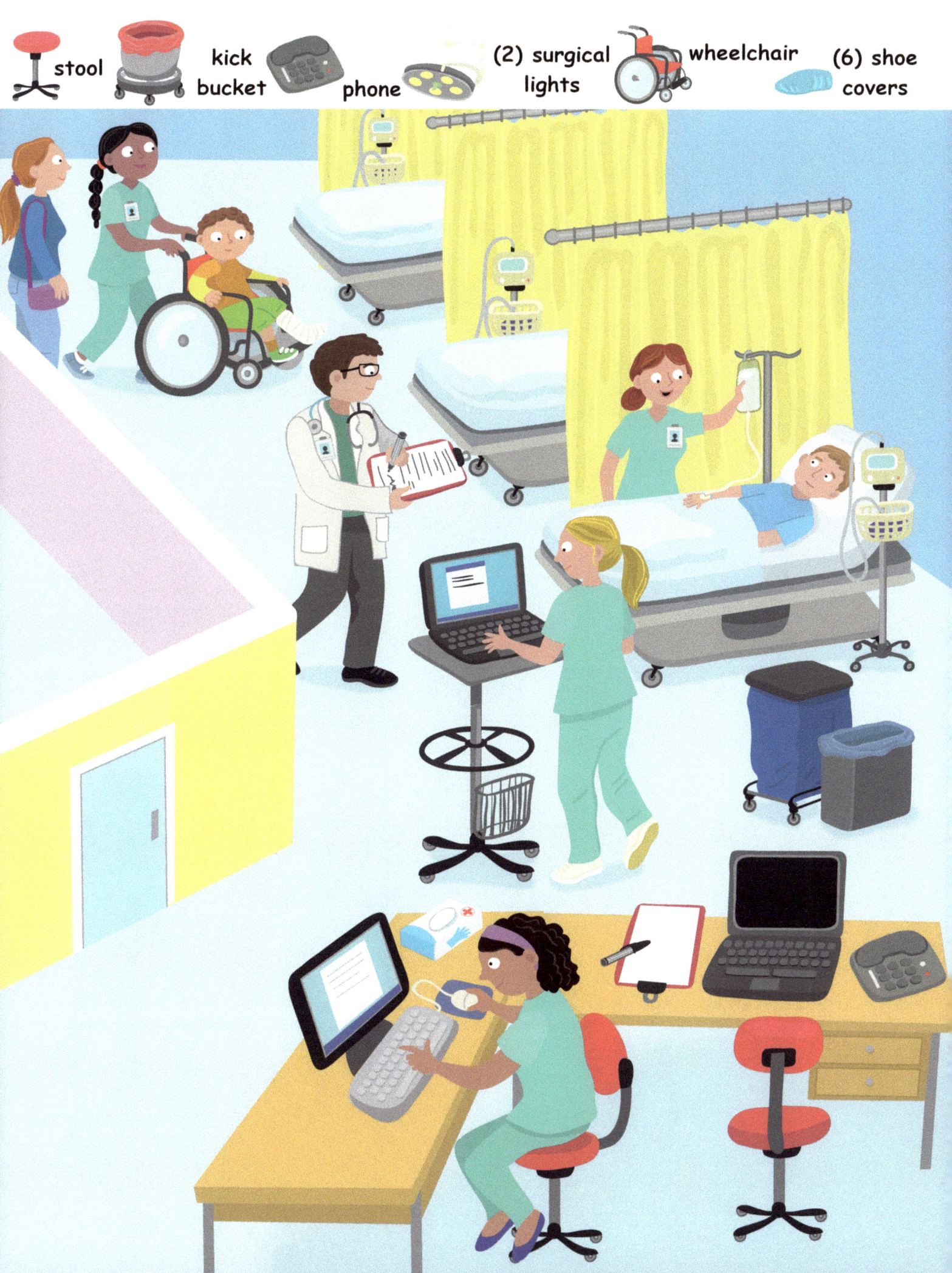

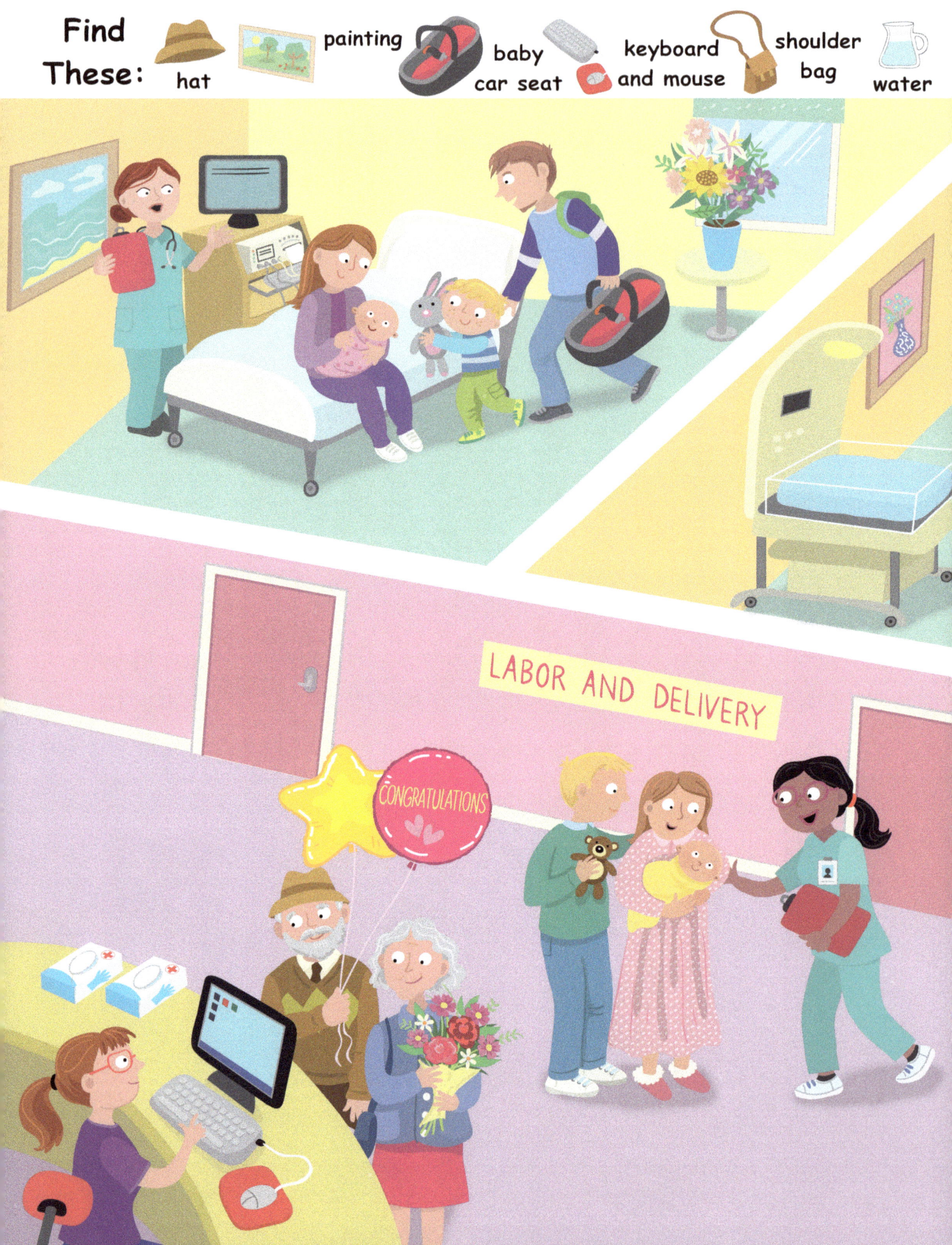

picture · exercise ball · baby warmer · bear · rocking chair · flowers

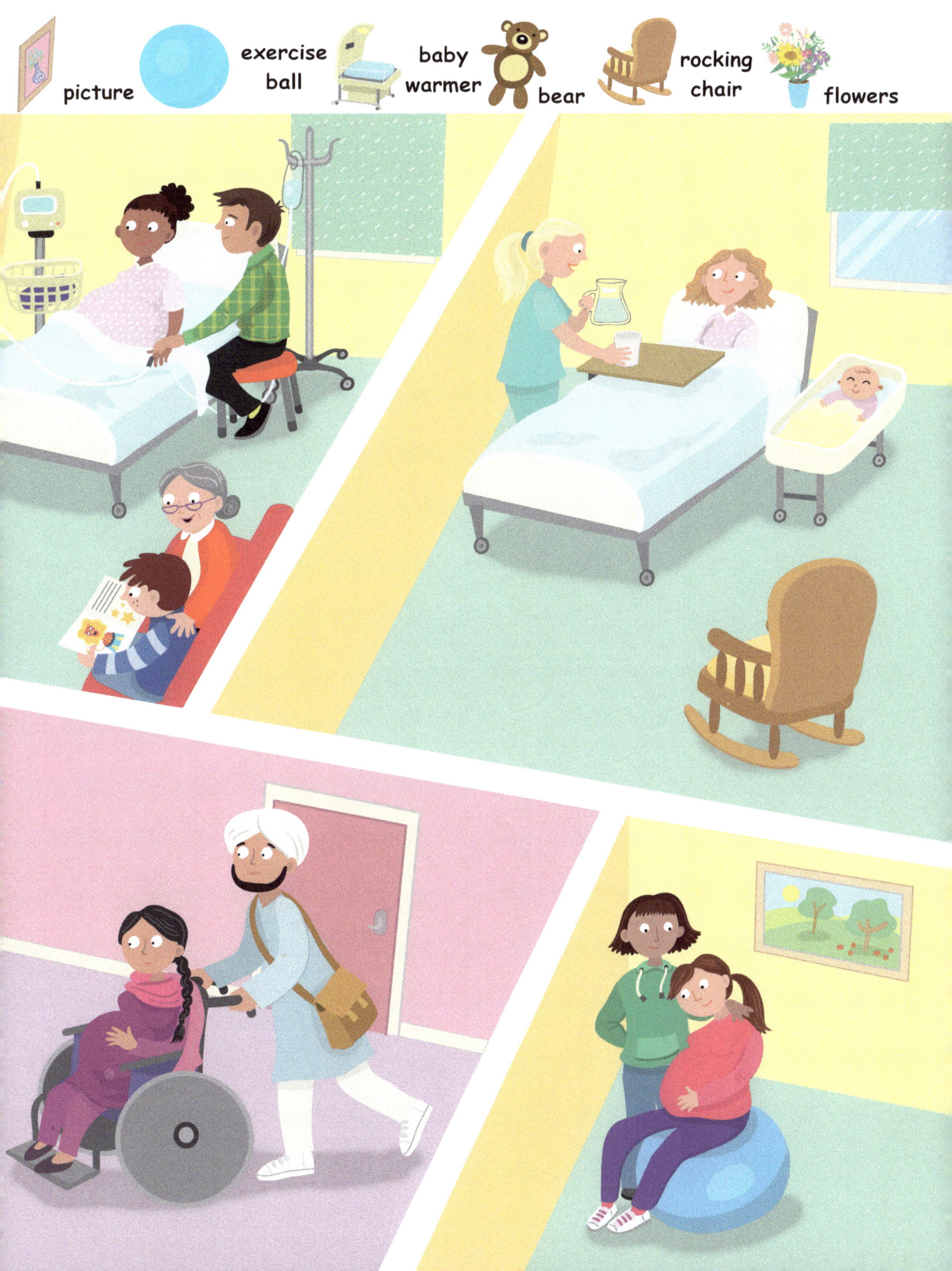

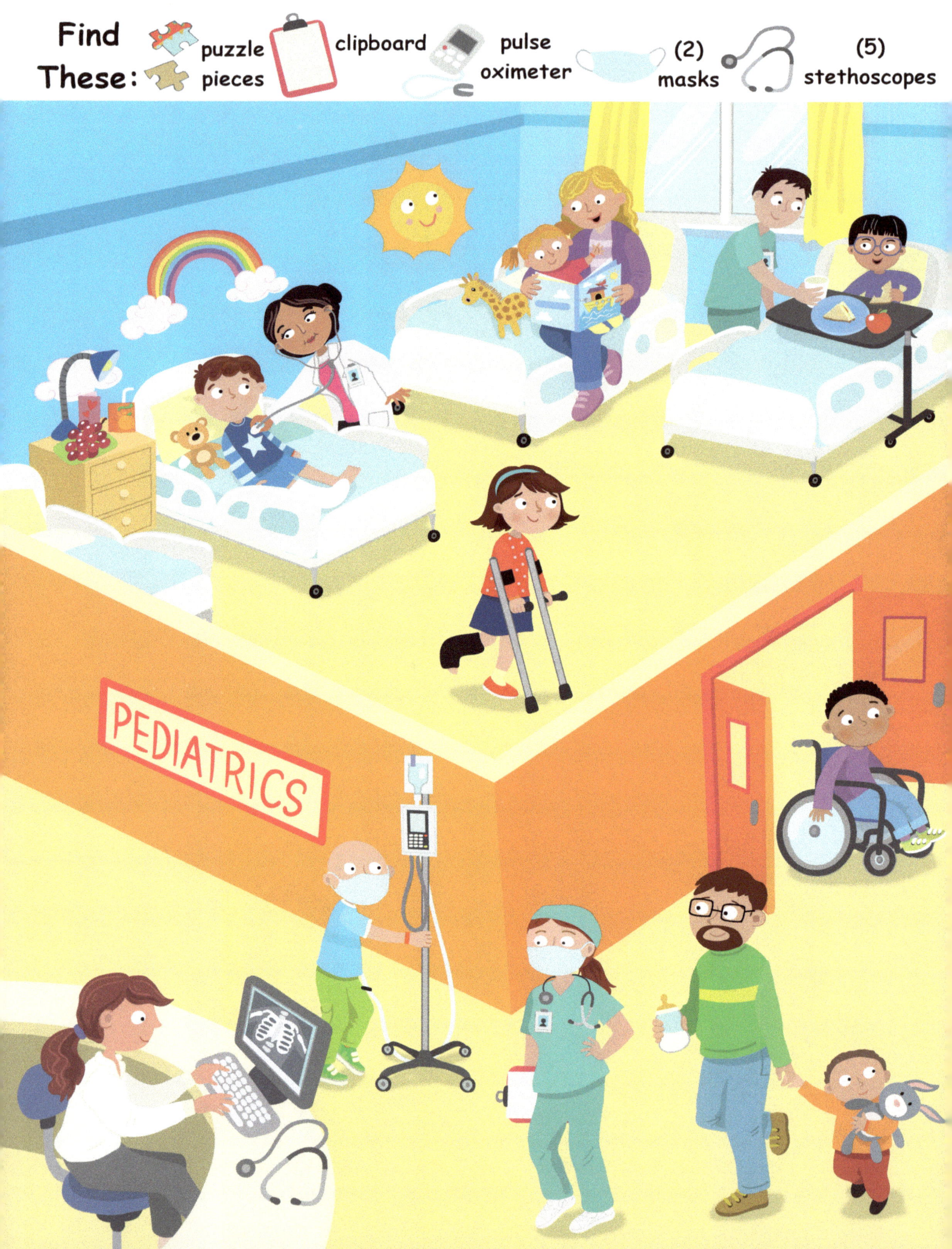

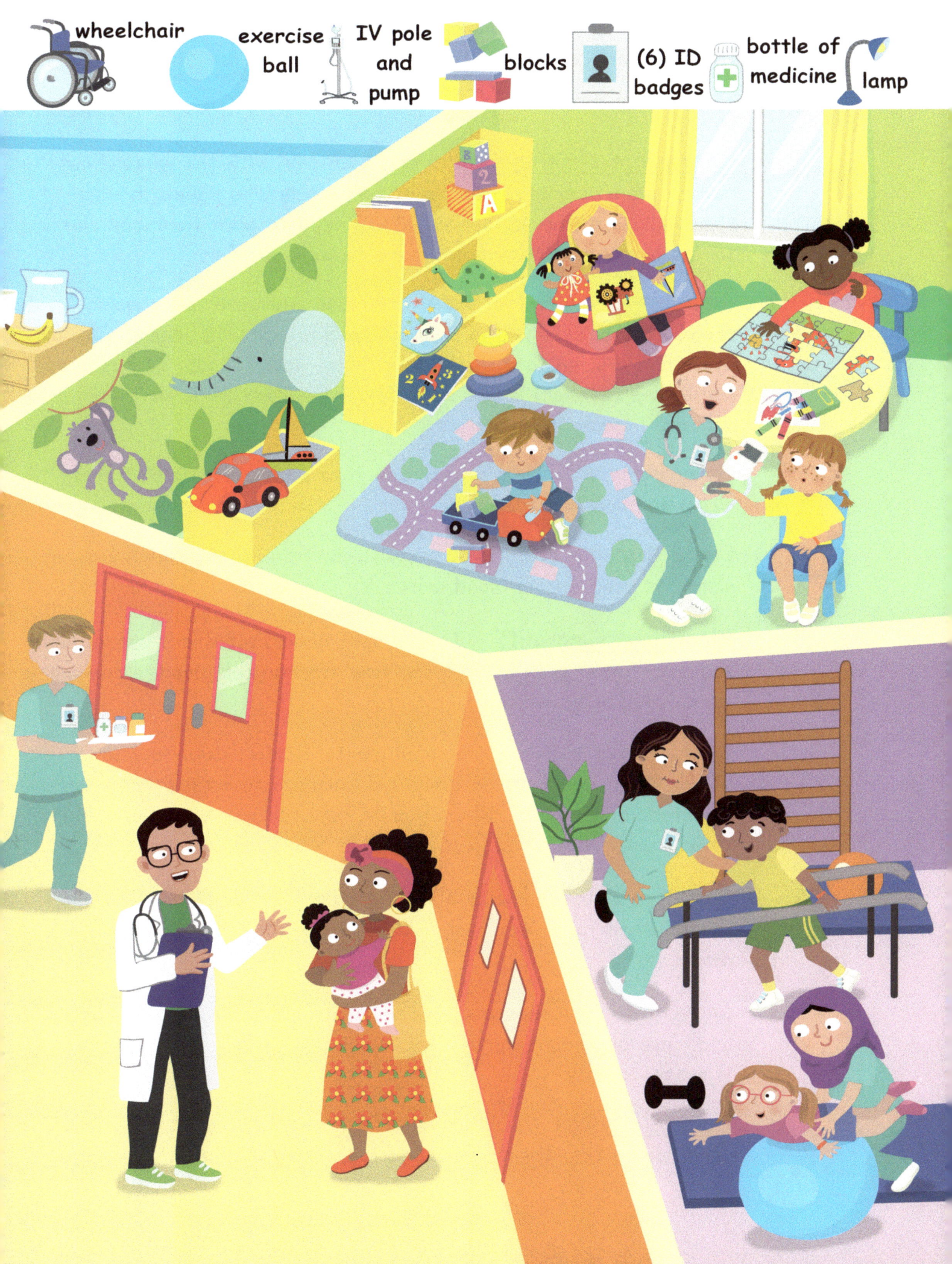

Glossary

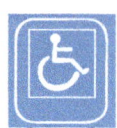
Accessible parking sign - This blue sign with the wheelchair means it's a special parking spot for people who have a harder time walking or moving around. They need to park their car closer to the hospital so they don't have to walk too far.

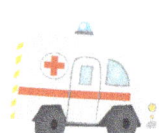
Ambulance - A special car that brings injured or very sick people very quickly to the nearest hospital. It has bright, flashing lights and a siren that makes loud "woo-woo" sounds. It has a bed (called a stretcher) in the back for the person to lie down and get help right away from the paramedics.

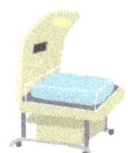
Baby warmer - It is a cozy bed that keeps brand new babies warm and comfortable.

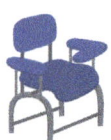
Blood drawing chair - A special comfortable chair with big armrests used during blood draws.

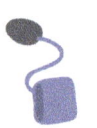
Blood pressure cuff - It is a soft band that wraps around and squeezes the arm briefly to see how strong your blood is pushing inside your blood vessels.

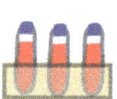
Blood tubes - These are small plastic bottles used to store blood. The tubes come in different colors, and each color is for different blood tests. When you or someone you know gets their blood drawn, the blood gets stored in blood tubes.

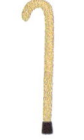
Cane - A walking cane is a special stick that helps people walk better when their legs feel wobbly or tired so they don't fall down.

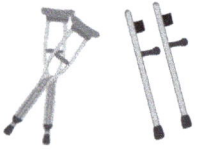
Crutches - Crutches are special sticks that help people stand up and move around when they hurt their leg or foot or when their legs feel wobbly.

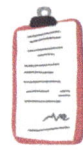
Doctor's notes - Doctors write down notes about the patient's condition to help them remember everything and see if they get better every day.

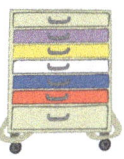
Emergency cart - It is a metal drawer on wheels that is full of special tools and medicines that doctors and nurses use when someone very sick needs help super fast.

Exercise ball - This is a big, squishy ball used for stretches and gentle, slow moves to help the body feel better and get stronger.

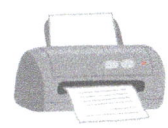
Fax machine - This machine very quickly sends and receives paper messages and photos from far away. It is like a super fast mail.

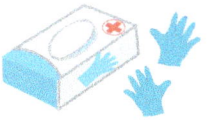
Gloves - Gloves help protect hands from germs.

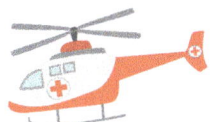
Helicopter - Medical helicopters can very quickly bring people who are hurt or very sick to the hospital. There is a small bed inside for the sick person to lie down and get help right away.

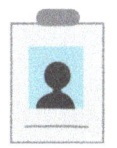
ID (identification) badges - Name tags for everyone who works in the hospital. It shows their picture, their name, and what they do.

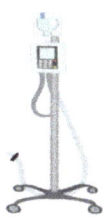
IV (intravenous) pole and pump - The IV pole is a tall metal stick on wheels at the bottom and hooks at the top for hanging medicine or fluids. The IV pump is a machine that delivers a set amount of medicine or fluid to the body through an intravenous catheter.

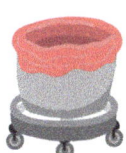
Kick bucket - A metal bucket on wheels used in the operating room to store used surgical cloths during a surgery. It is gently moved with the foot in the operating room to keep things clean and organized.

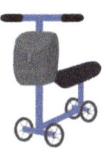
Knee scooter - This scooter is helpful when someone hurts their ankle or foot and cannot walk for a while. They can rest their hurt leg on the seat and use the other foot to scoot around.

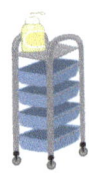 **Lab (laboratory) cart** - Cart on wheels used to store supplies. This cart has a bottle of hand sanitizer on top to help people clean their hands.

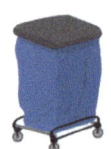 **Linen bin** - It is a big laundry basket on wheels for used towels, blankets, and sheets so they can get washed.

 **Mask** - Masks are worn over the nose and mouth to stop germs from spreading.

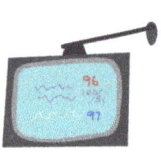 **Monitor** - Medical monitors help doctors and nurses see patients' heartbeat, blood pressure, breathing, and temperature so they can help patients feel better. The monitors sometimes make beeping noises when the patients might not feel well.

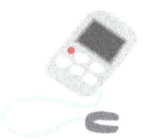 **Pulse oximeter** - A small finger hugger that checks the heart rate and how much oxygen is in the blood. It does not hurt.

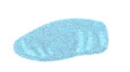 **Shoe covers** - These covers keep the shoes clean during surgery.

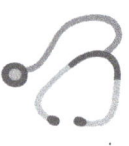 **Stethoscope** - A cool medical tool that some doctors and nurses wear around their necks. It is used to listen to the heart, lungs, and abdomen (or tummy). It may feel a little cold on the skin, but it won't hurt.

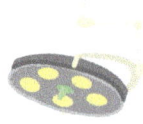 **Surgical lights** - These are big and super bright lights above the operating table that help surgeons see well during surgery. There's usually a handle in the middle of the light for the surgeons to move it around.

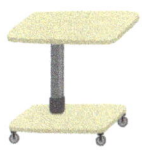
Table on wheels - These are used like any other table and can be easily moved from one place to another.

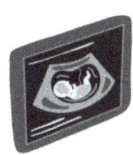
Ultrasound picture - Ultrasound uses a camera-microphone (called a probe) to see and listen to the inside of the body, like the heart, the tummy, or a tiny baby inside a mom's belly. The pictures can be shown on a monitor or be printed.

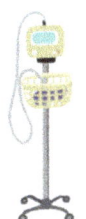
Vital signs monitor - These monitors have wheels and can be easily moved from one place to another. They also help doctors and nurses see patients' heartbeat, blood pressure, oxygen level, and temperature so they can help patients feel better. The monitors sometimes make beeping noises to alert the doctors and nurses when the patients might not feel well.

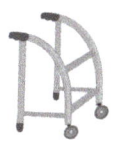
Walker - It is a metal frame with legs and wheels that help people walk better when their legs feel tired or wobbly.

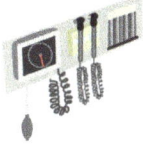
Wall station - This is a wall tool shelf that doctors and nurses use to check patients' blood pressure, their eyes, ears, nose, and throat. It is usually on the wall in a doctor's office.

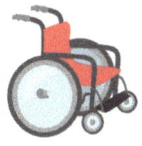
Wheelchair - A chair that rolls. It can be used when someone has trouble walking or moving around.

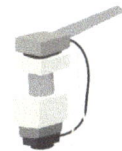
X-ray machine - A special camera that takes pictures of the inside of the body, like bones and organs.

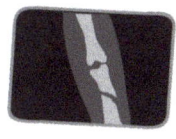
X-ray picture - A special picture that shows the inside of the body, such as bones and organs.

It's time to explore some more!

Can you find these busy hospital workers:

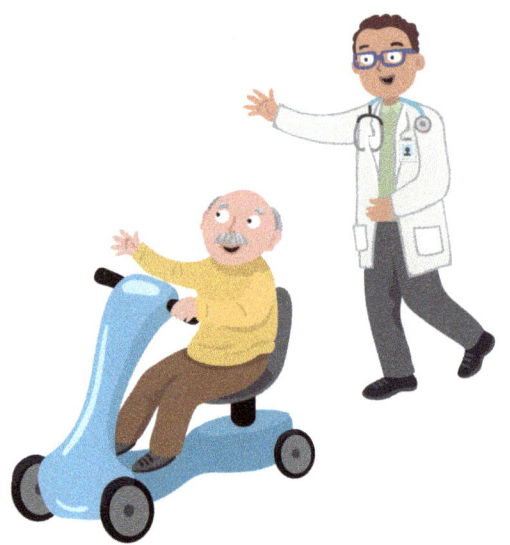

A doctor is waving goodbye to his patient and wishing him a speedy recovery.

The medical resident (a doctor in training who is supervised by a licensed doctor) is telling her patient when she should come back to the hospital for a follow-up appointment.

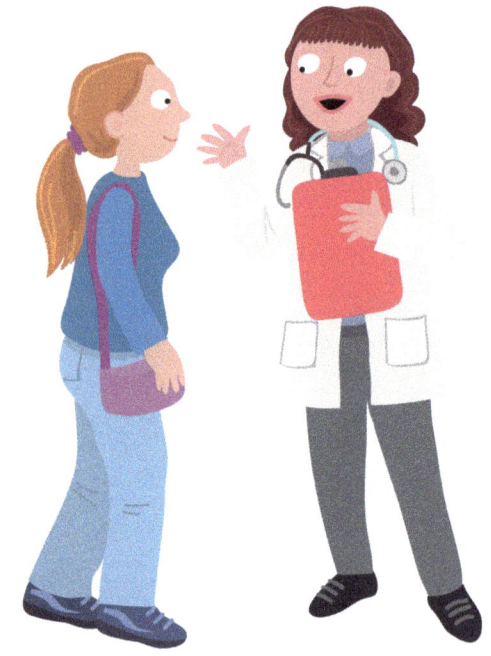

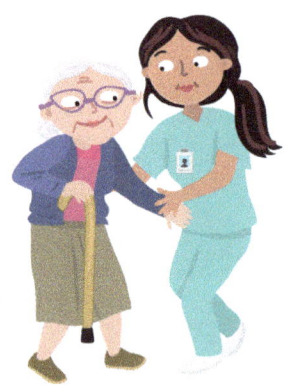

A nursing assistant is helping this elderly lady walk to her car.

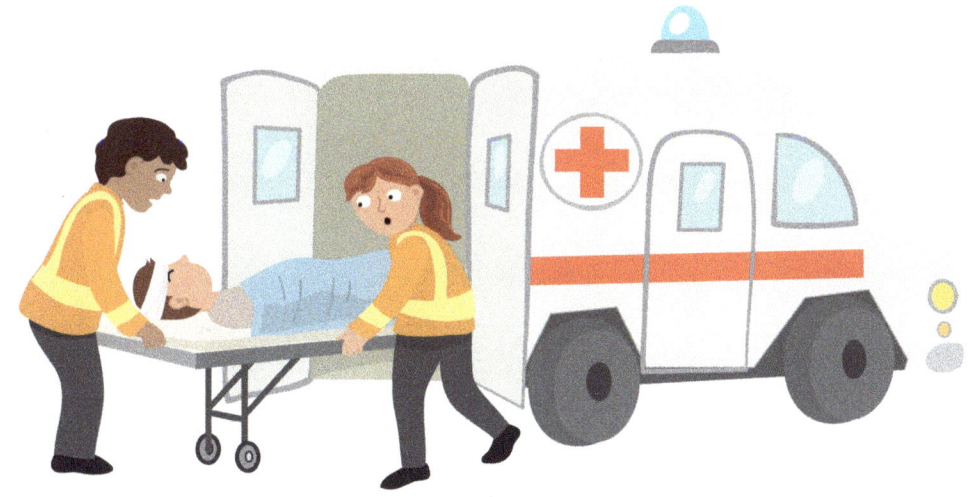

The paramedics are bringing an injured patient to the hospital in an ambulance.

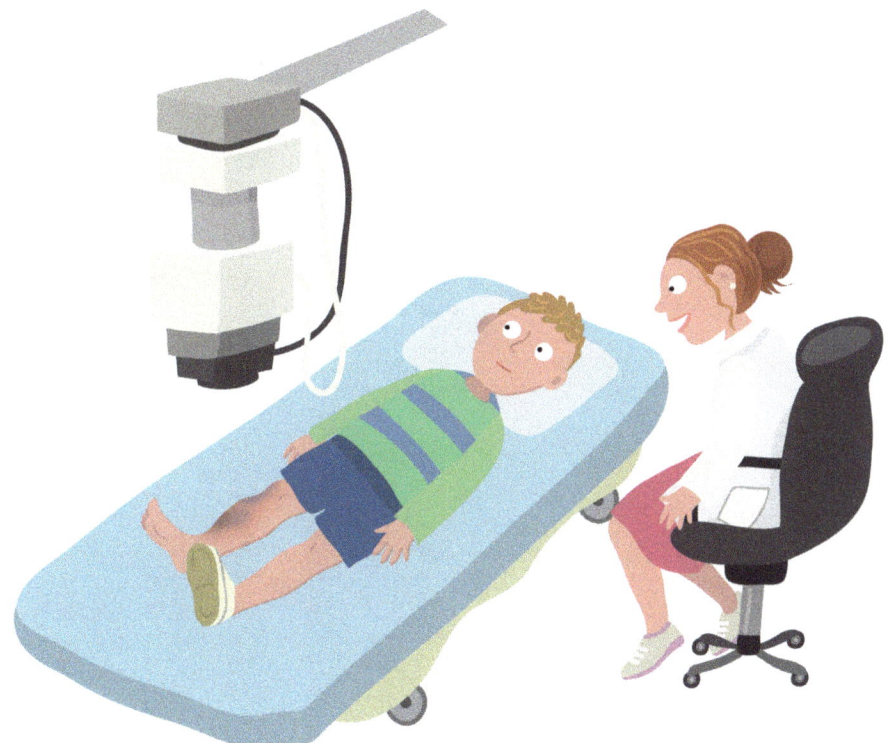

A radiologist (picture doctor who sees the inside of the body by looking at photos taken by machines) is making sure the boy is comfortable before more pictures are taken of his injured leg.

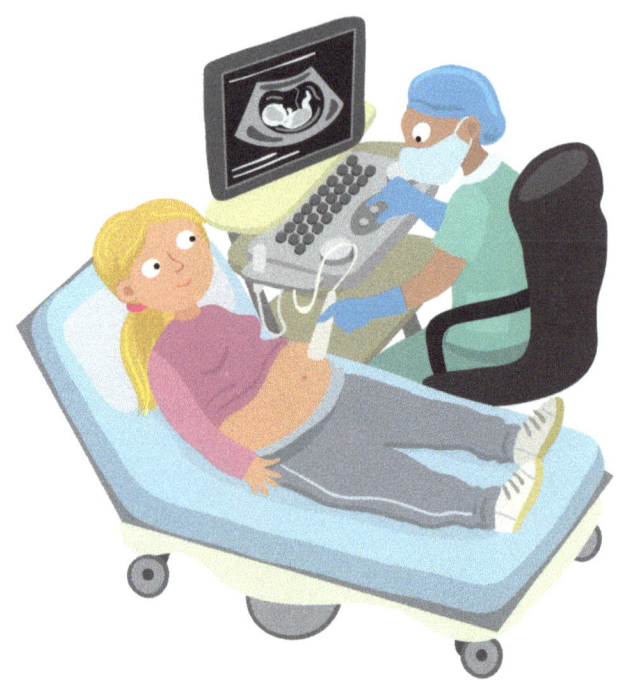

An ultrasound technician is using the ultrasound camera-microphone, called a probe, to help this mother see her growing baby inside her tummy.

A phlebotomist is drawing blood from the girl's arm for her doctor to see how healthy she is on the inside.

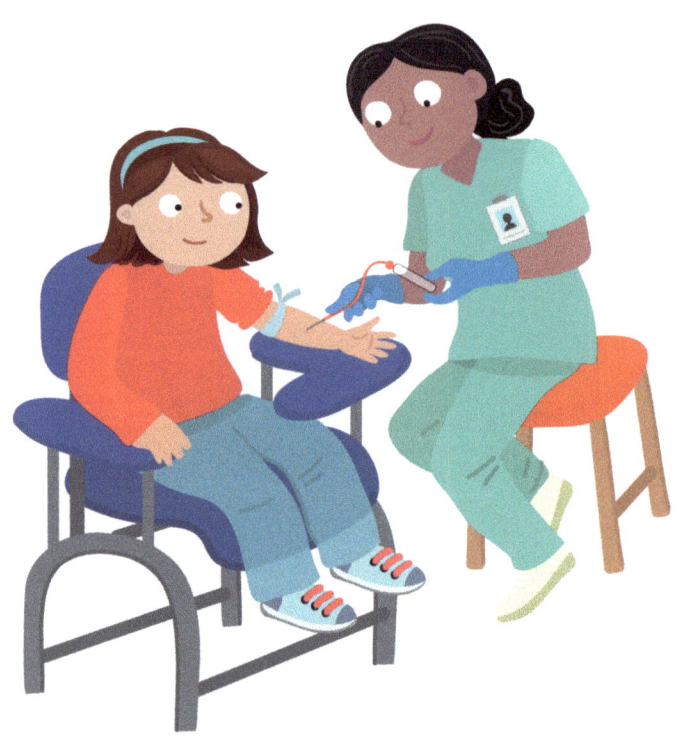

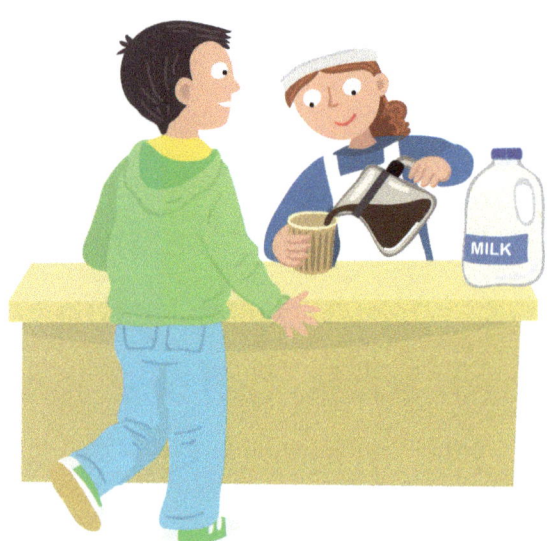

The cafeteria worker is pouring a cup of coffee for the visitor.

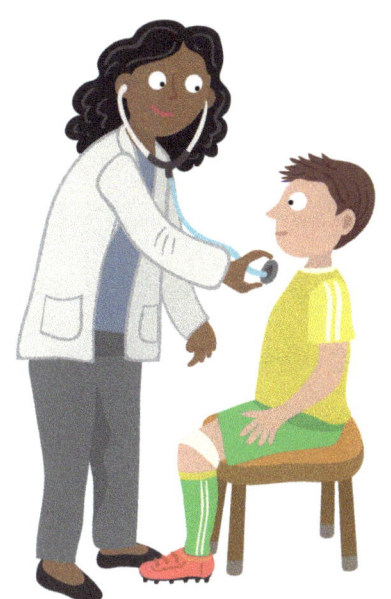

A medical student (supervised by a licensed doctor) is learning how to become a better doctor by listening to her patient.

An X-ray technician is bringing a portable (mobile) X-ray machine to his next patient.

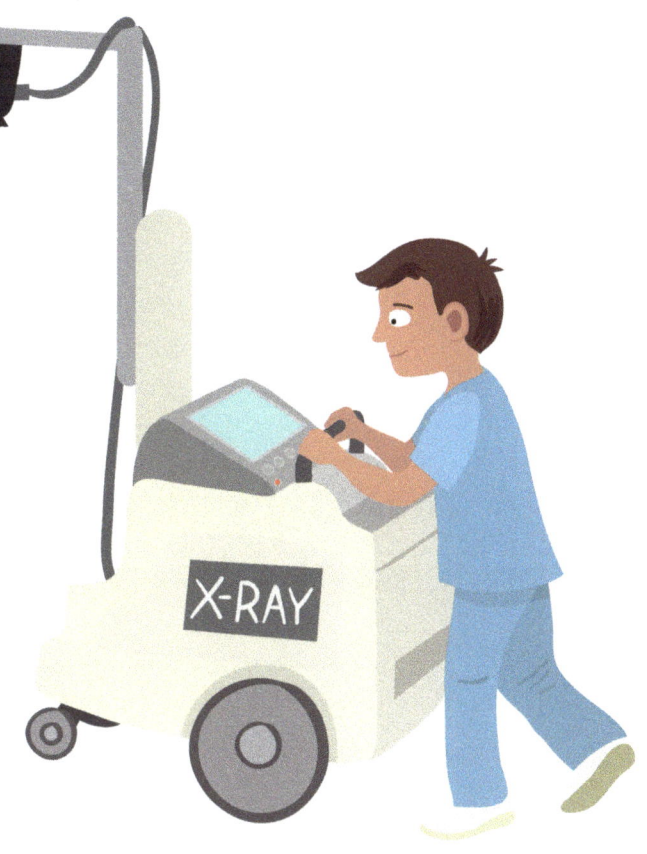

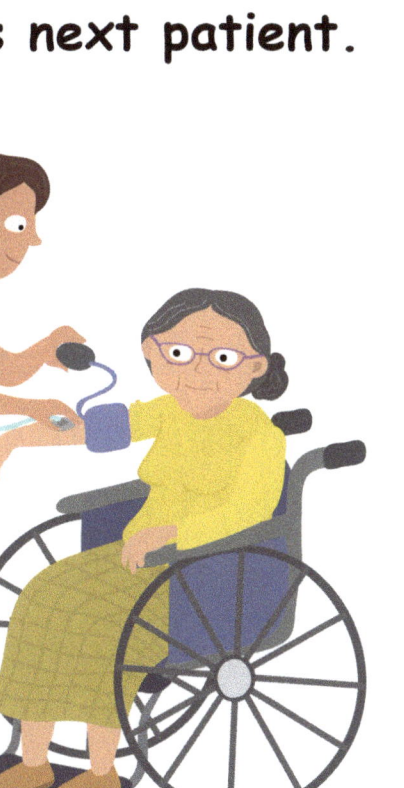

The nurse is checking the patient's blood pressure to make sure she is feeling better.

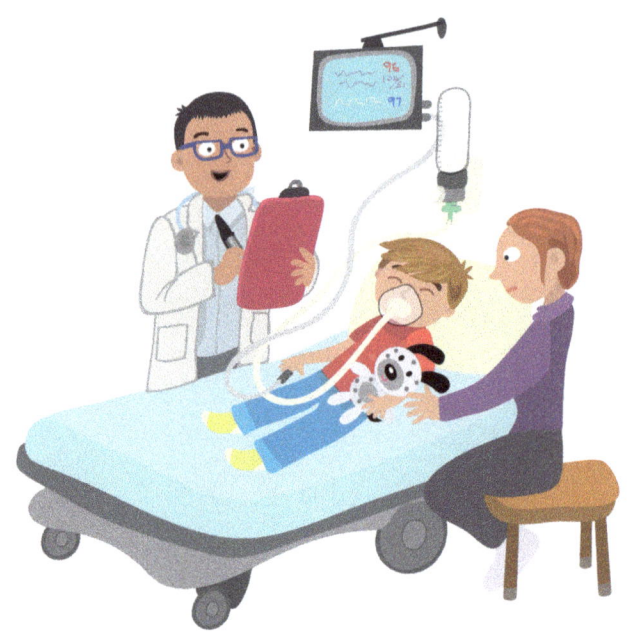

The respiratory therapist is checking up on the little boy to make sure he is more comfortable and his breathing is better.

A food service worker is bringing the boy his lunch.

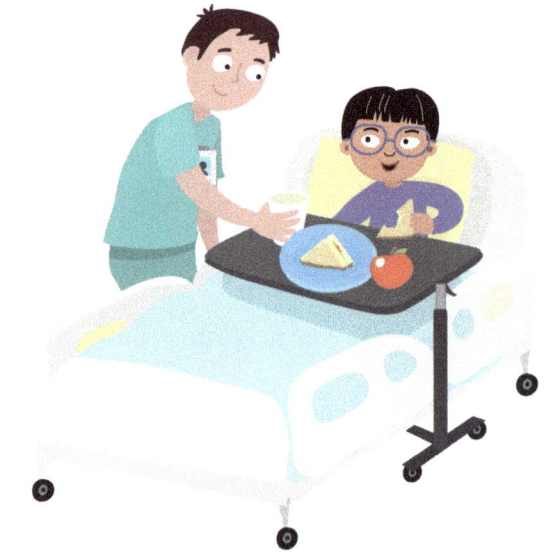

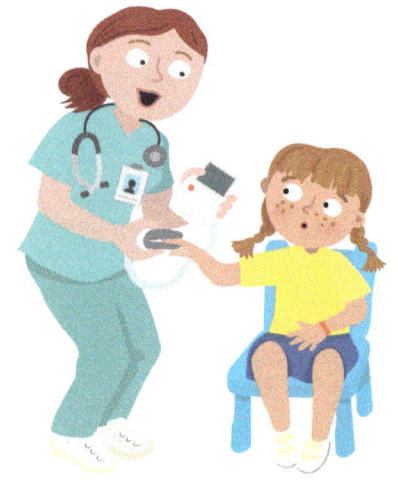

The medical assistant is checking the girl's oxygen level in her blood with a pulse oximeter.

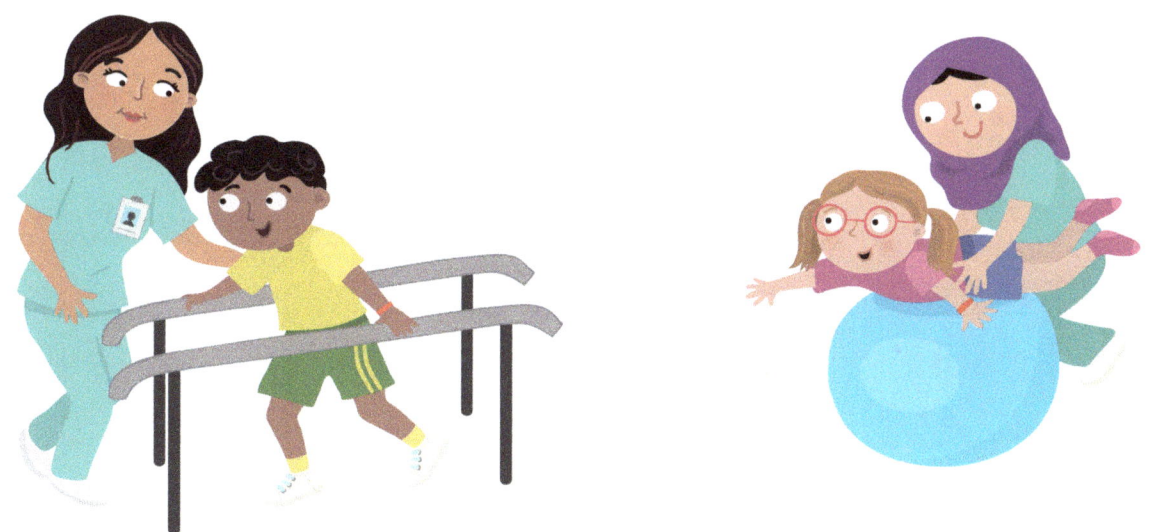

Physical therapists teach patients how to correctly move their body to feel better and get stronger.

A janitor is cleaning up a spill on the floor to keep the hospital clean.

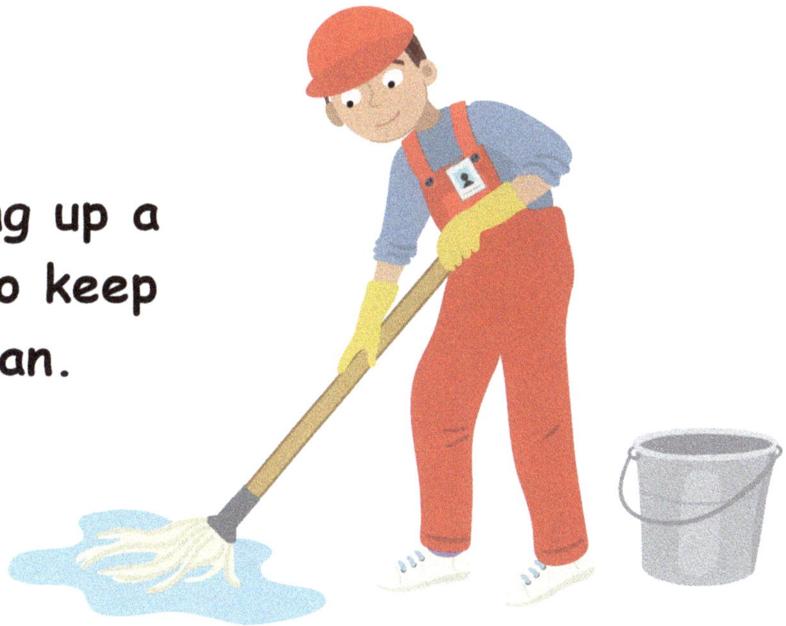

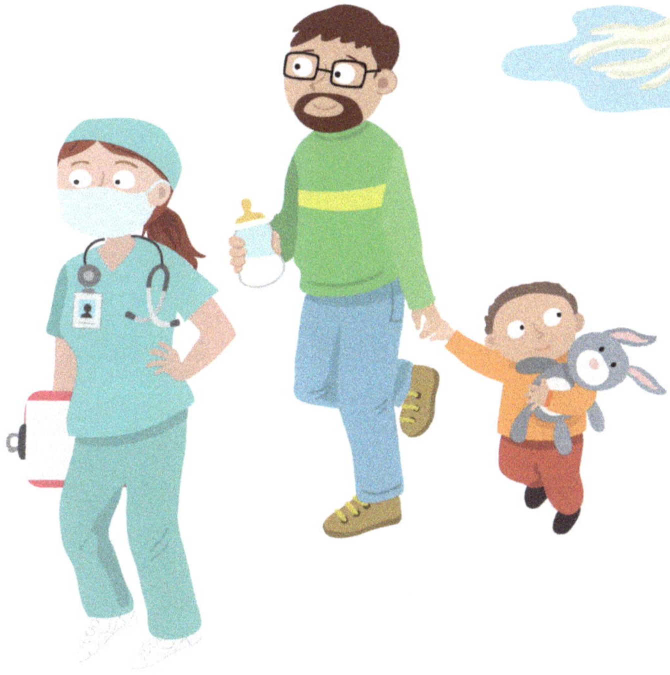

A child life specialist provides support and resources to children and their families.

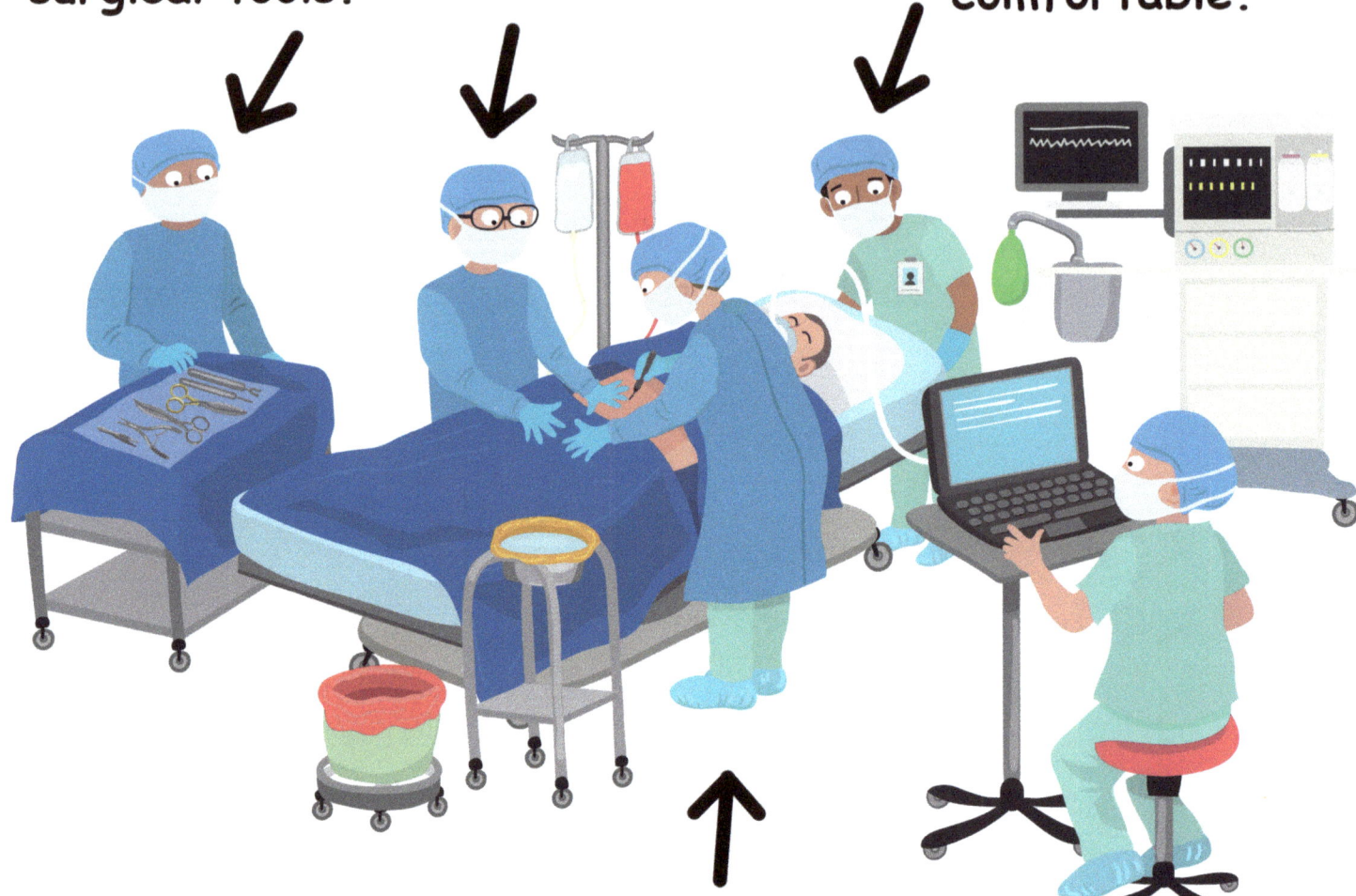

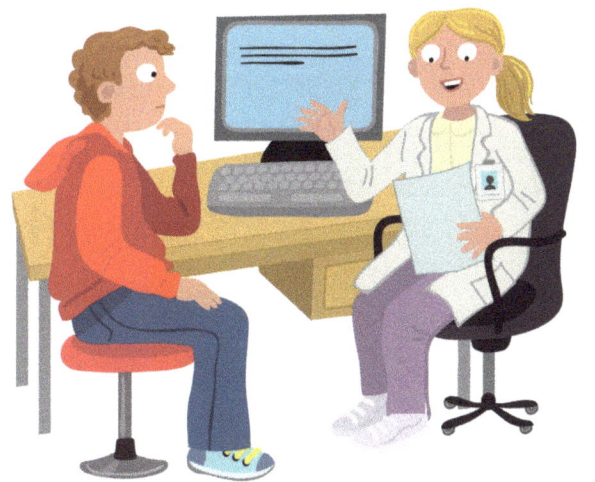

A physician assistant helps doctors see and treat more patients.

The nurse is writing a note (called a progress note) in the patient's chart about how the patient is doing.

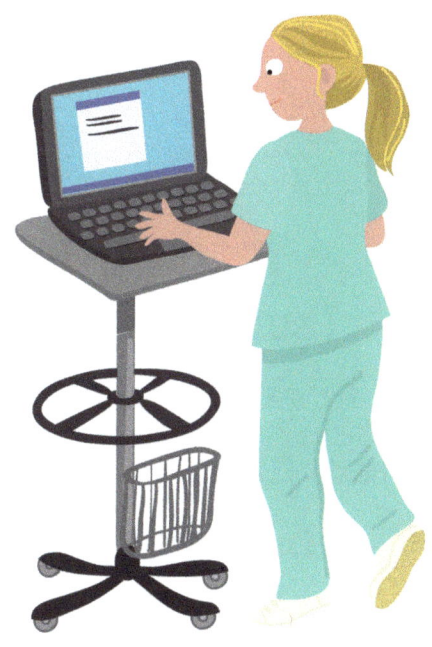

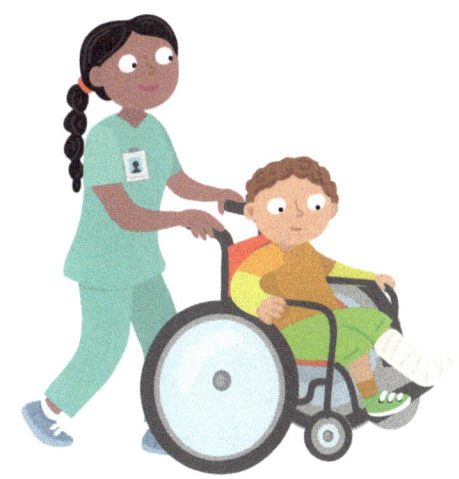

A licensed vocational nurse (LVN) helps transport this boy to his surgery.

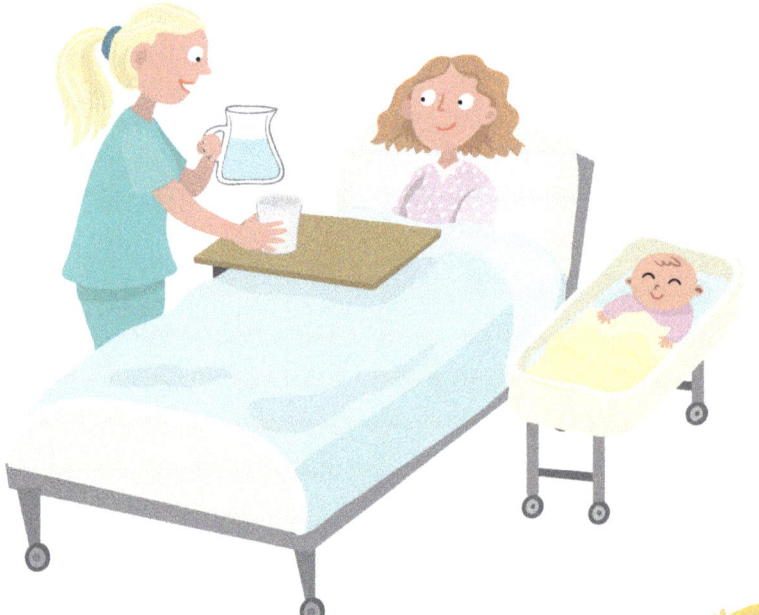

A nurse's aide is bringing some water to a mother with a new baby.

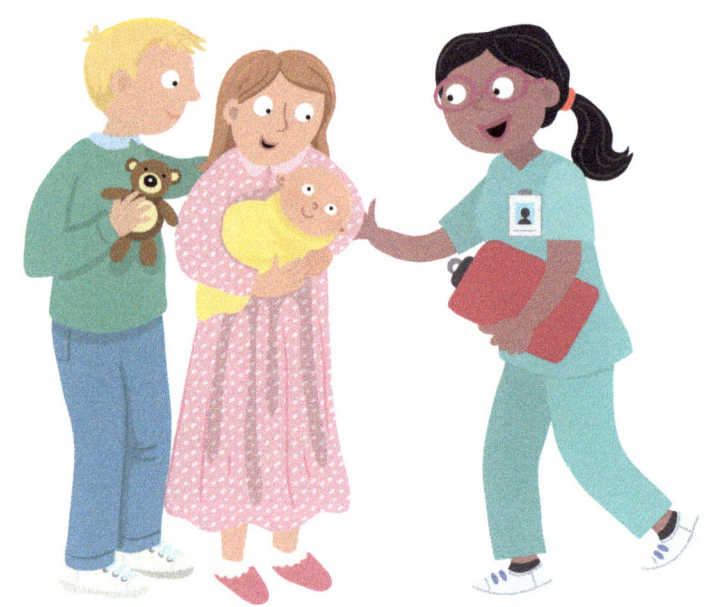

A medical intern (supervised by a licensed doctor) is learning to become a better doctor.

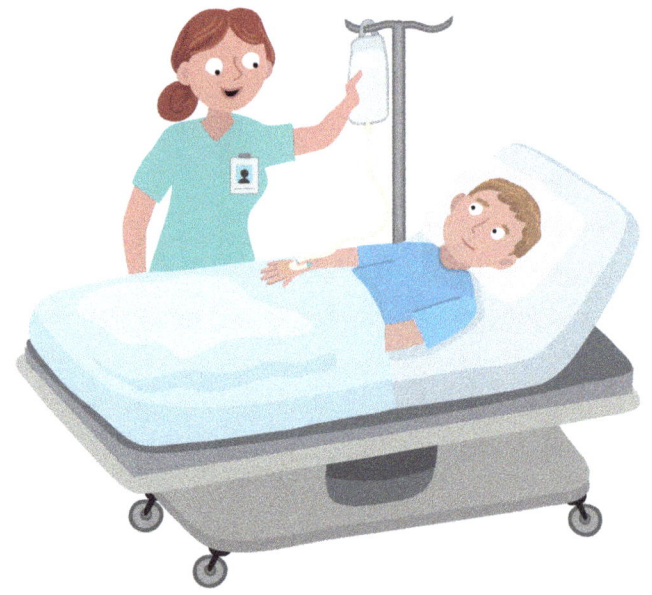

The perioperative nurse is getting the patient ready for surgery.

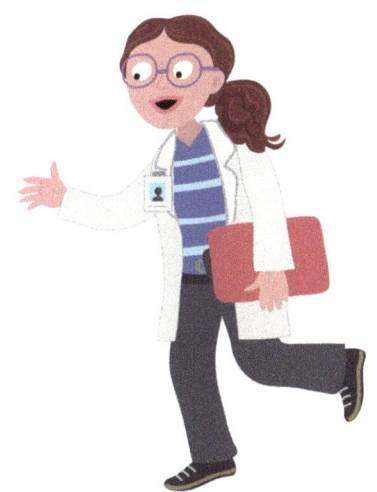

A doctor is walking quickly to see her next patient.

The blood laboratory aide is calling in the next patient for blood draw.

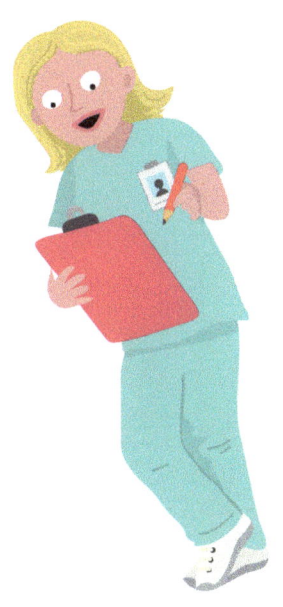

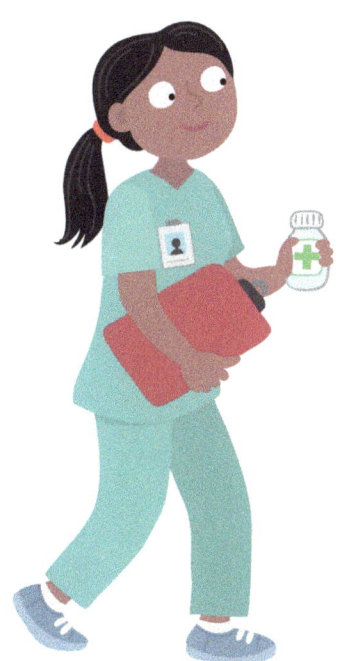

A medical runner is quickly bringing a bottle of medicine to a patient in a different part of the hospital.

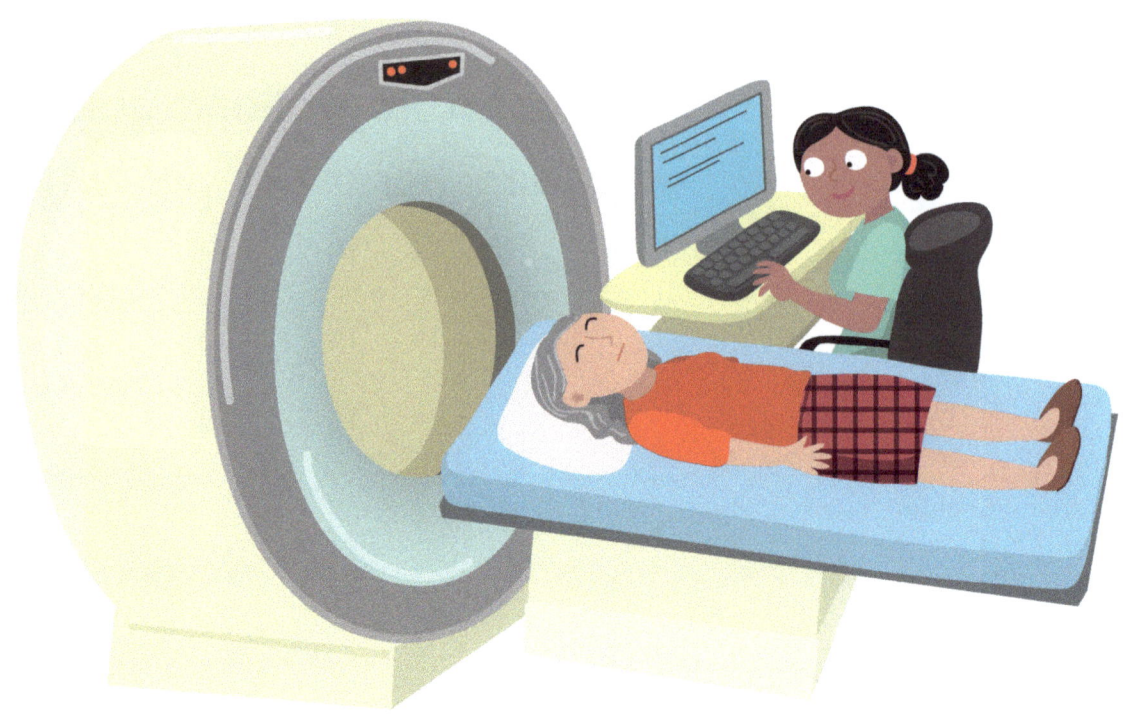

A CT (Computed Tomography) technologist operates the CT scanner to help see the different organs and tissues inside of the patient's body.

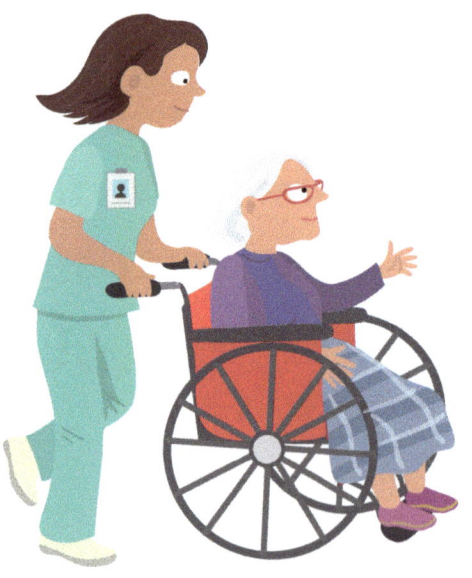

A patient transporter is taking this woman to her car outside the hospital.

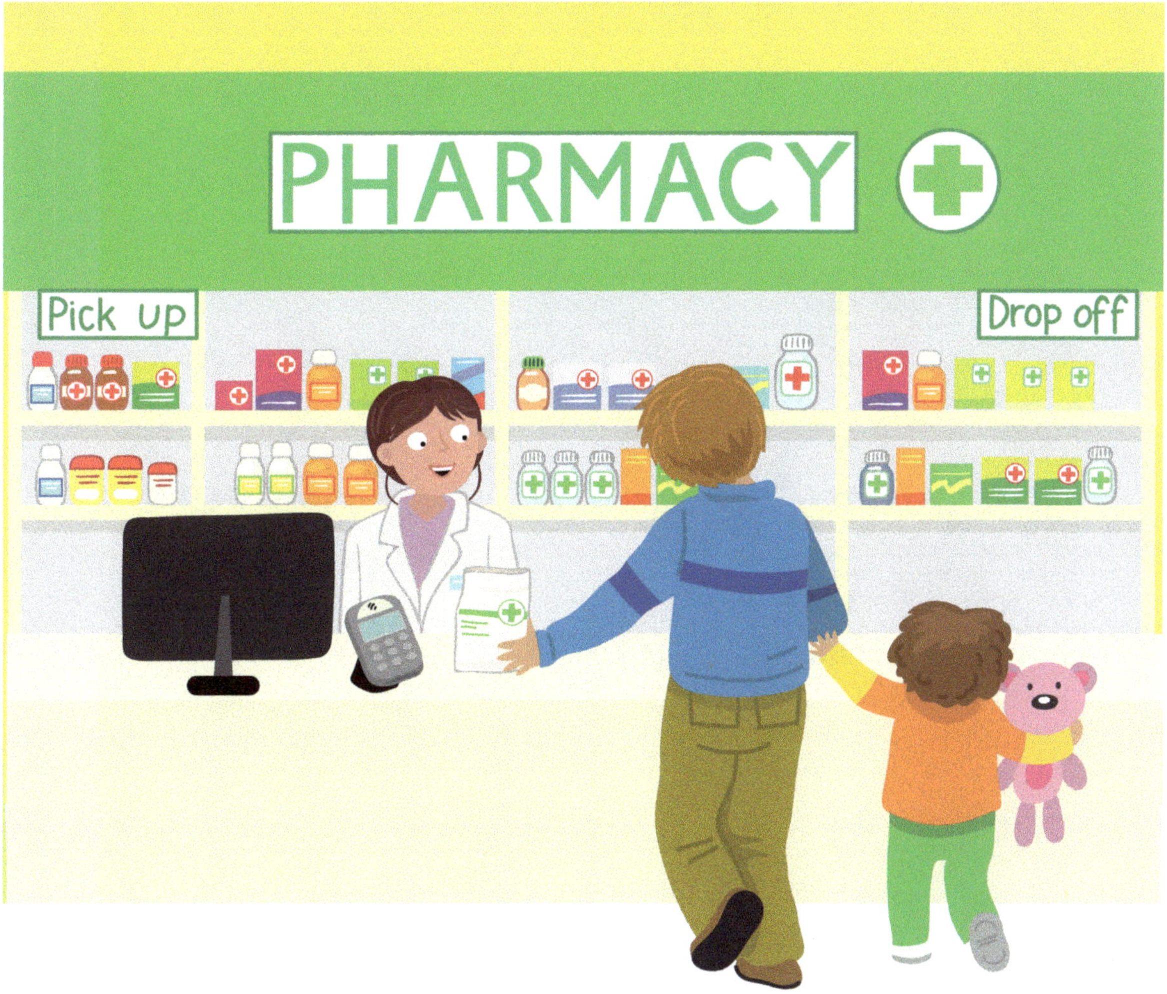

The pharmacist is knowlegeable about medicines and makes sure patients get the correct medicine to help them get better.

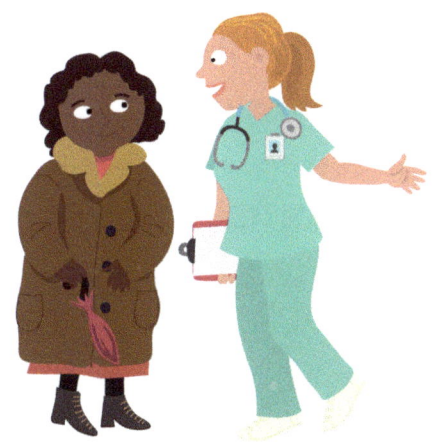

A nursing student (supervised by a licensed nurse) is learning how to become a better nurse.

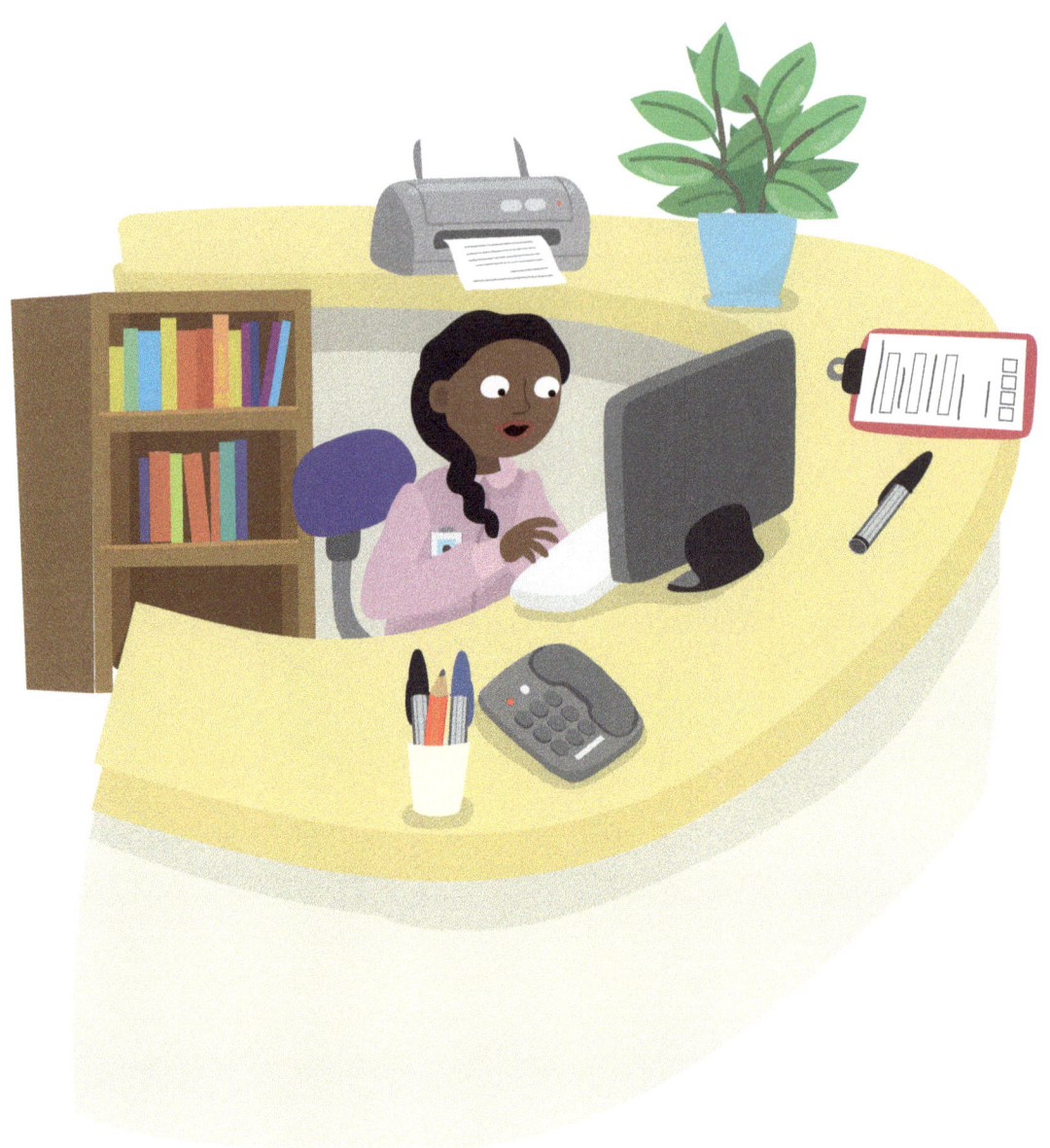

The hospital receptionist usually sits at a special desk near the entrance of the hospital, and they are there to help everyone with their questions.

There are also other receptionists who work at different parts of the hospital.

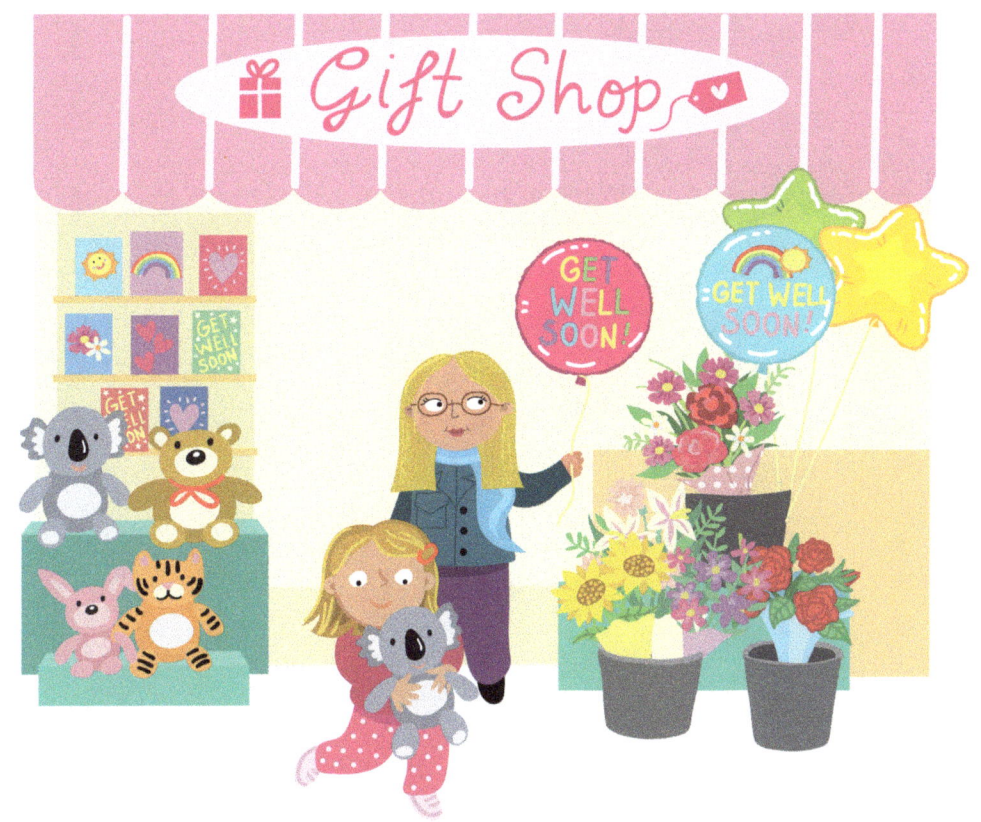

A gift shop worker works in the hospital's little store to help visitors pick out balloons, flowers, stuffed animals, or other gifts to cheer someone up.

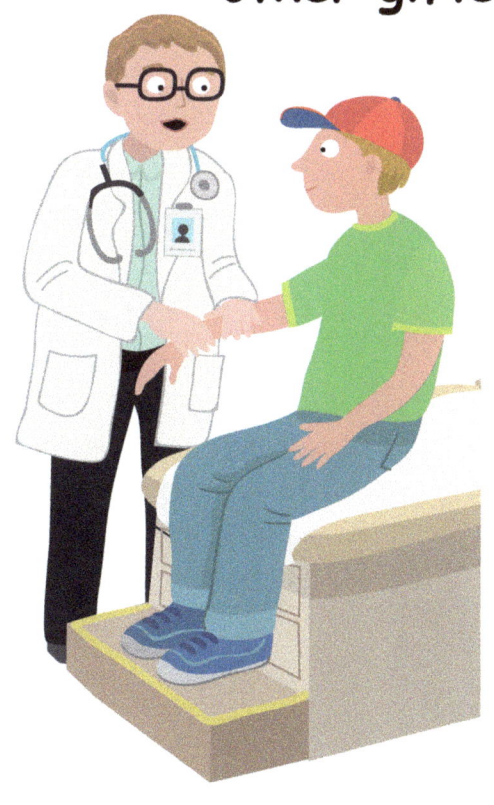

The doctor is examining the patient's arm to make sure it has healed and that the patient is feeling better.

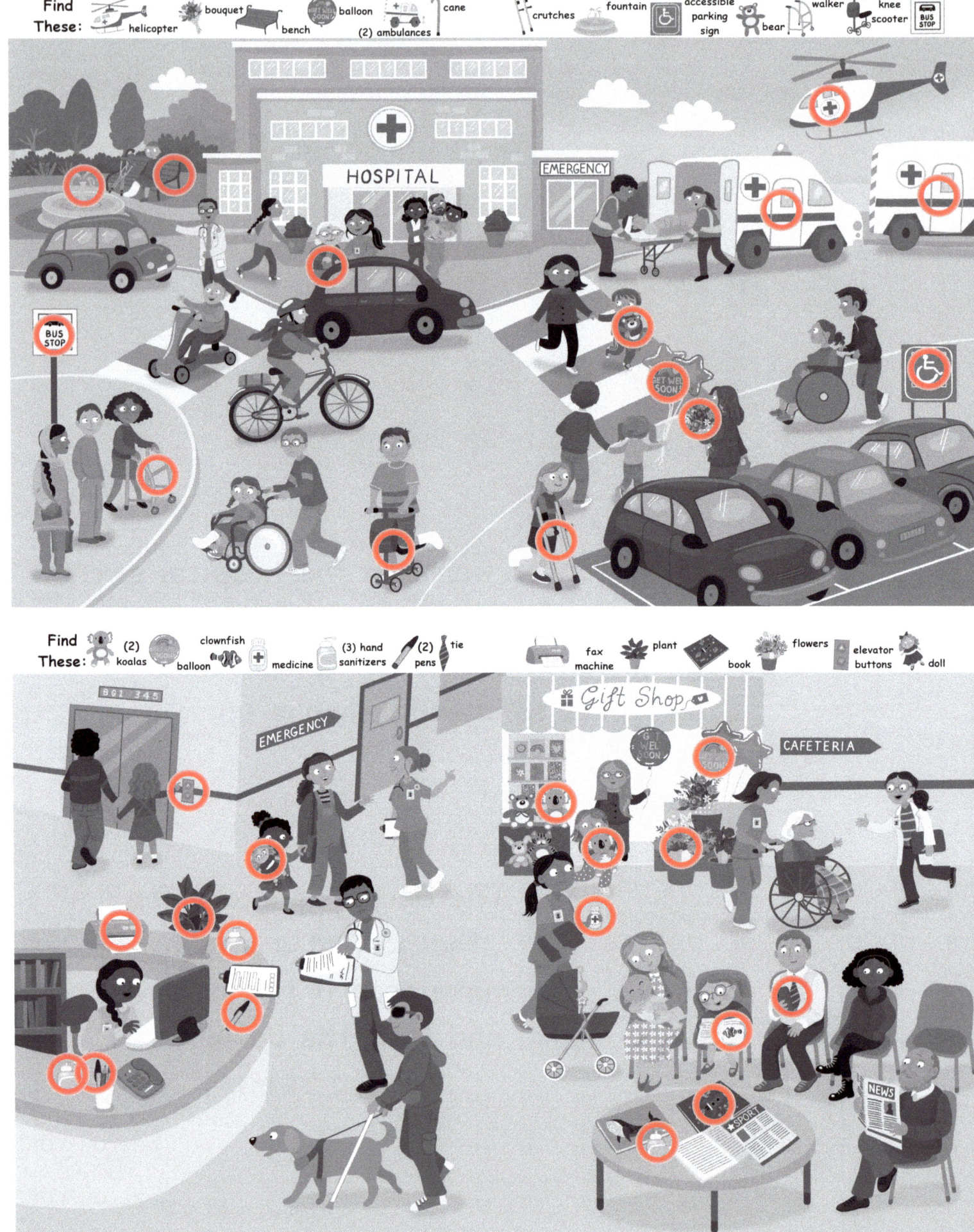

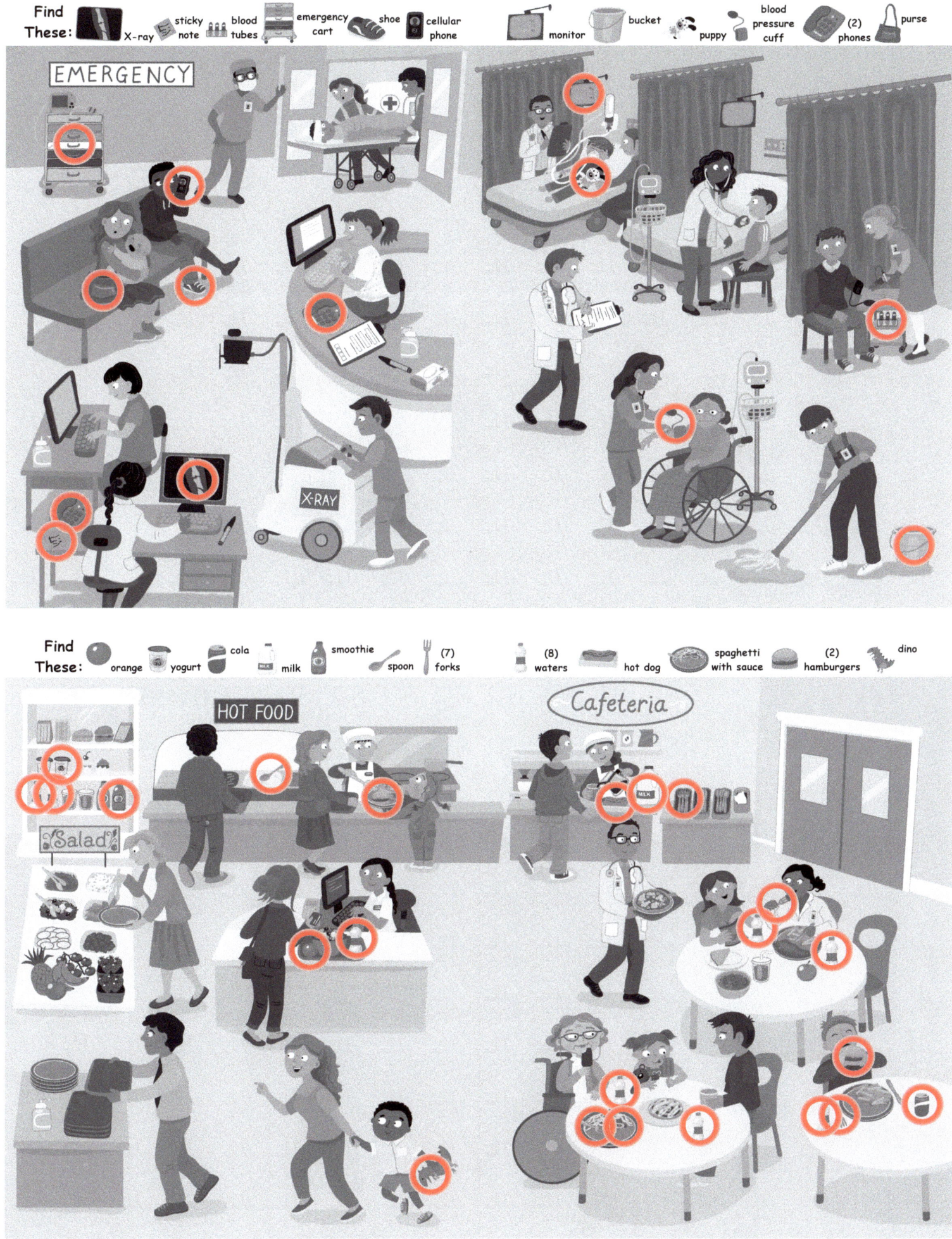

Find These: cap · book · bear · sink · cellular phone · (3) wall stations · shoe · newspaper and book rack · (2) linen bins · backpack · (4) boxes of gloves · beanie

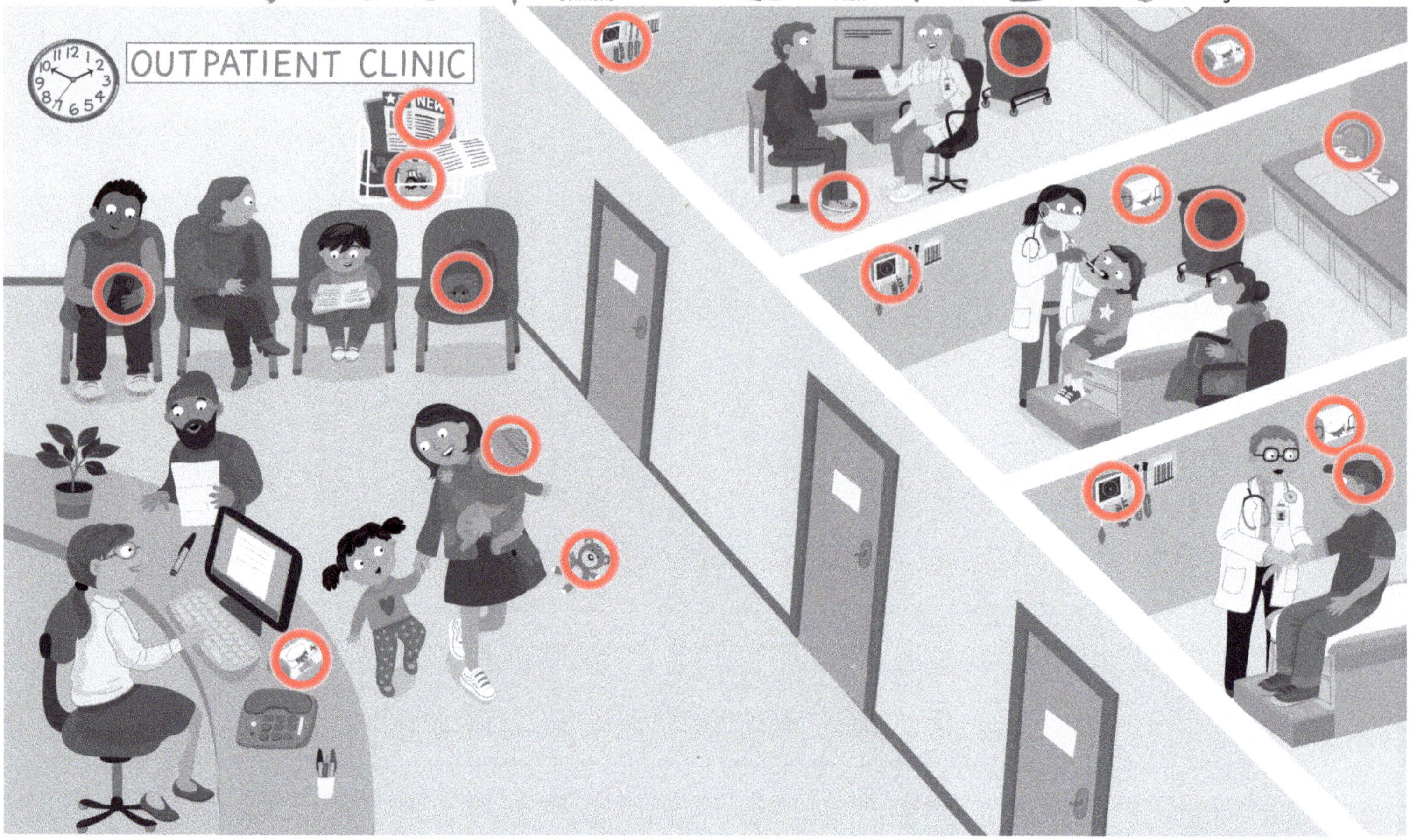

Find These: (2) stools · a bag of medicine · (2) boots · (2) lab carts · payment machine · computer · (3) boxes of medicine · medicine in a bottle · (2) tables on wheels · (3) blood drawing chairs · backpack · purse

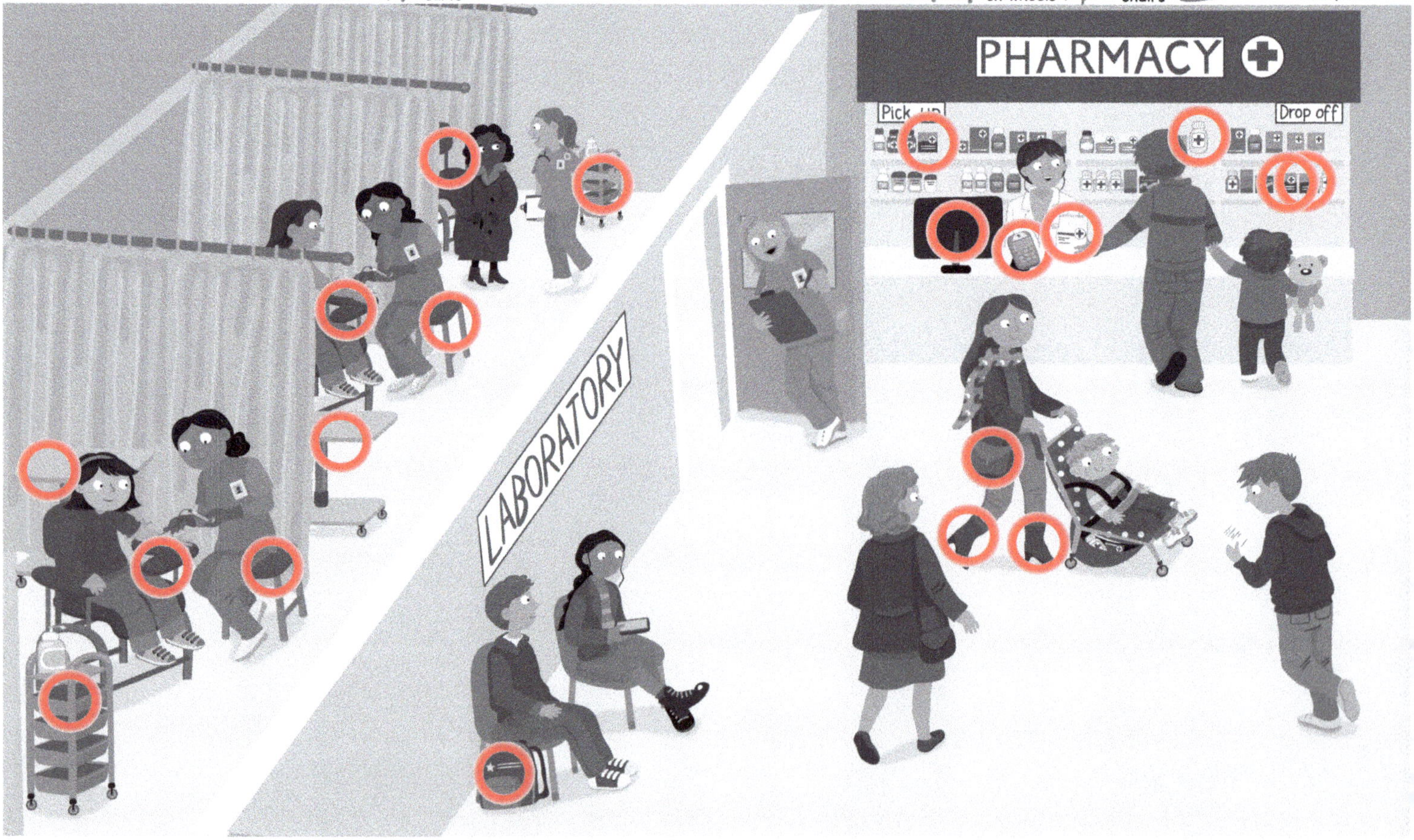

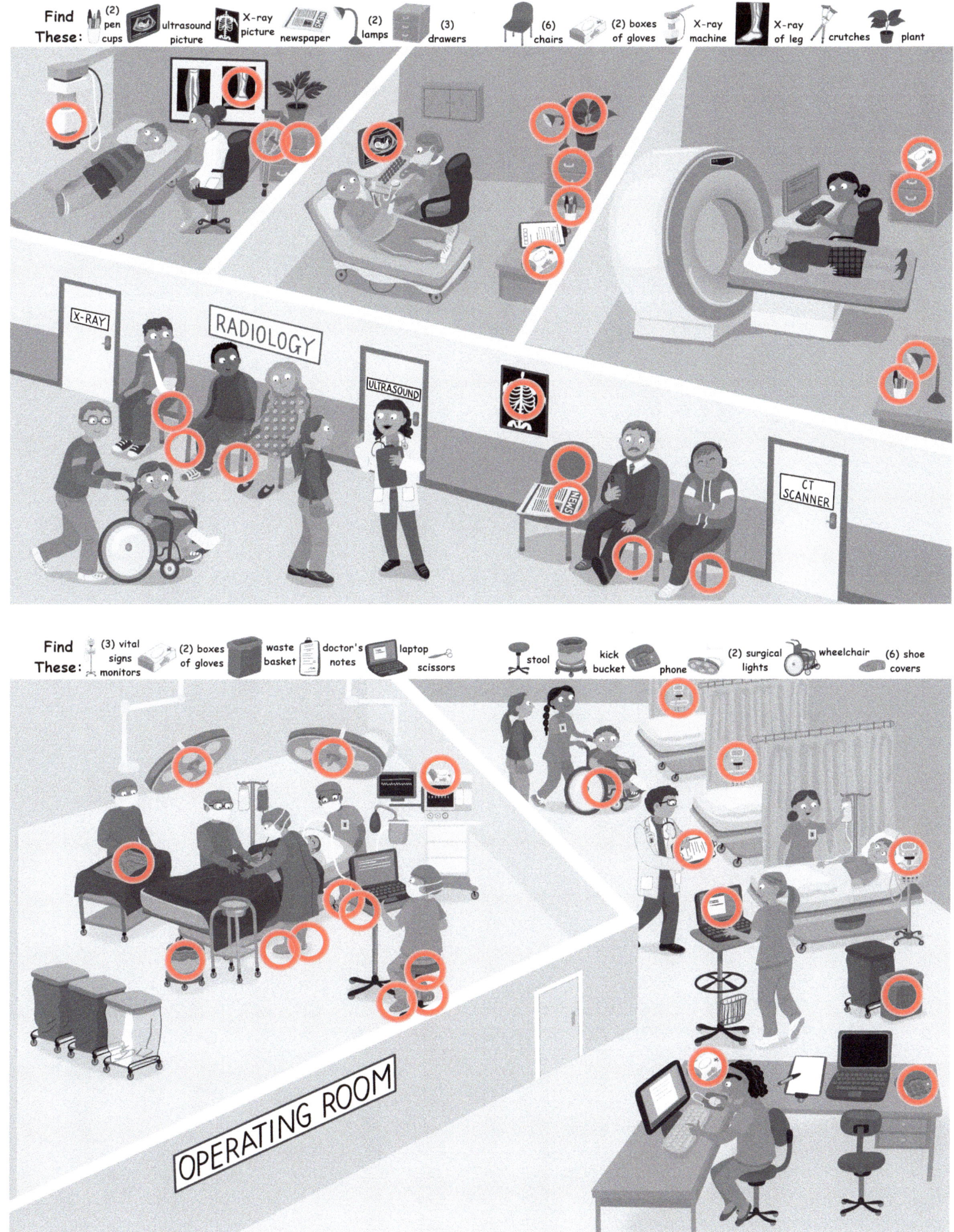

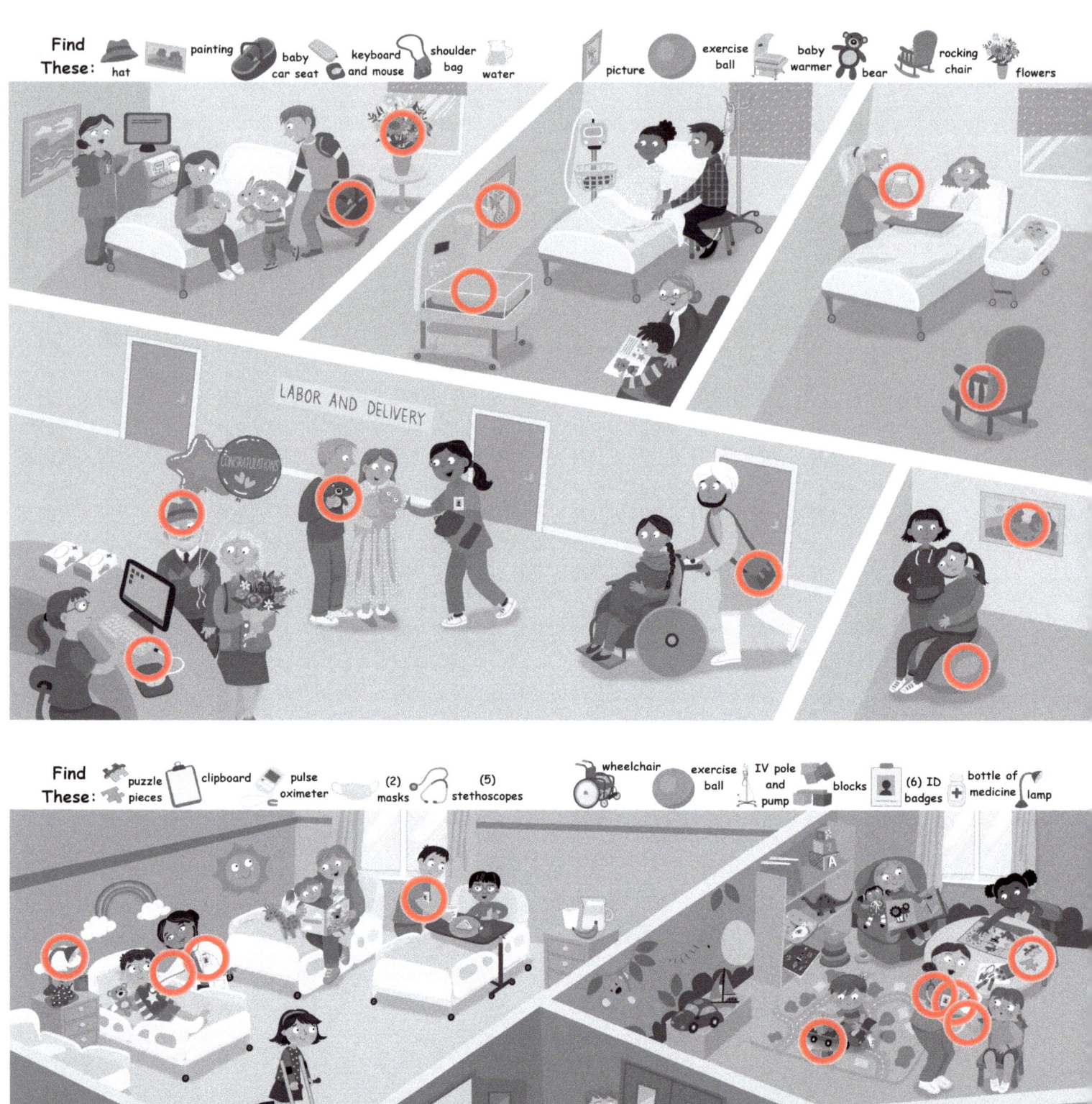

Did your little one enjoy this book?
If so, I would love to hear about it!

www.amazon.com/gp/product-review/B0F5N6NRXQ

For other book titles, please visit:

www.fzwbooks.com

To connect with the author:

email: books@fzwbooks.com

facebook/instagram: @FZWbooks

More books by the author

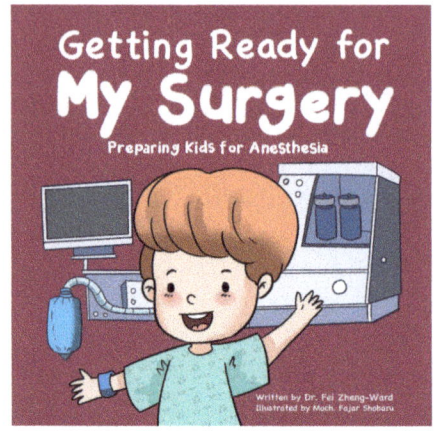
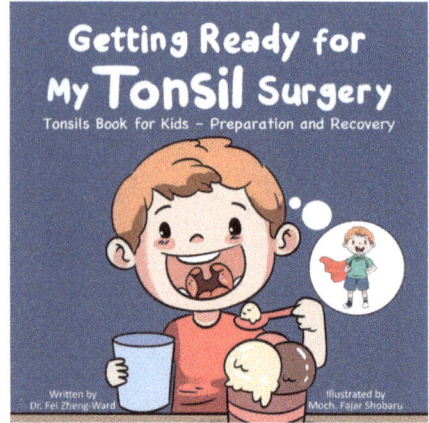
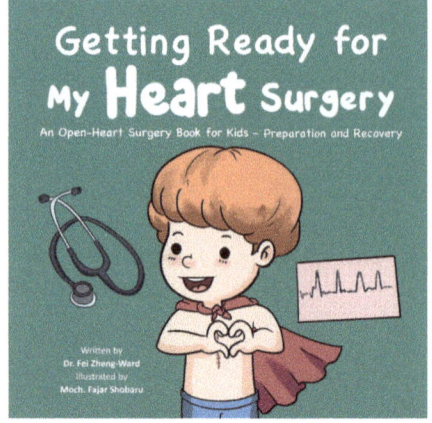
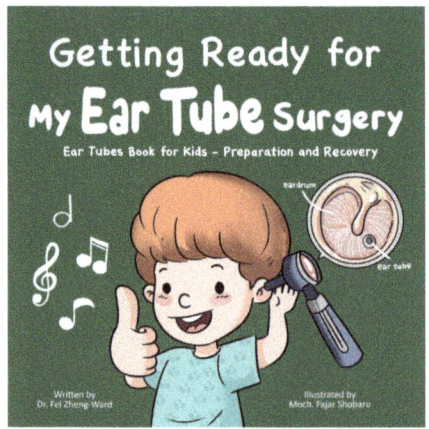
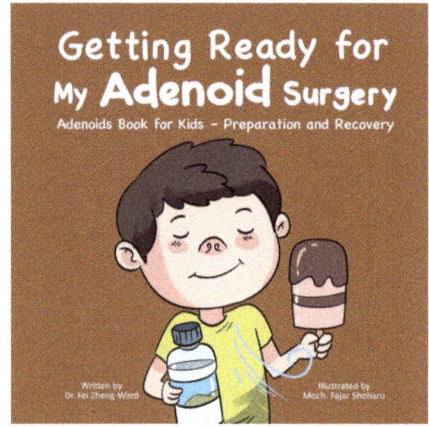
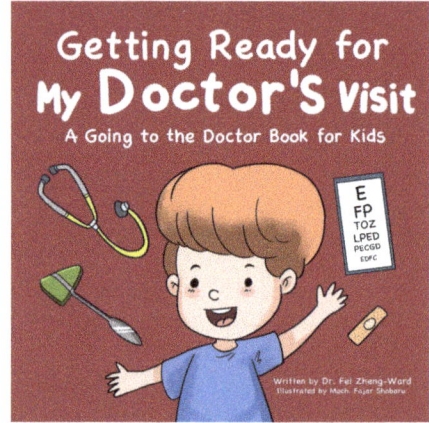
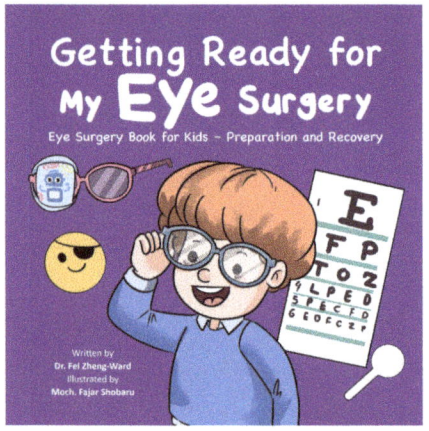
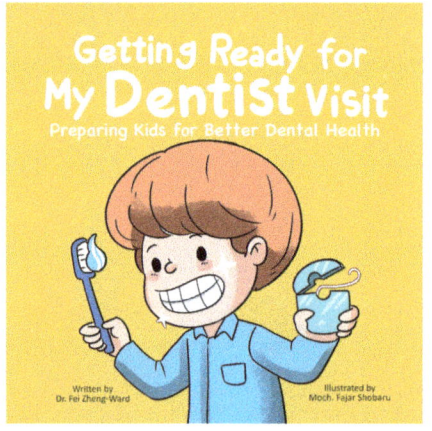
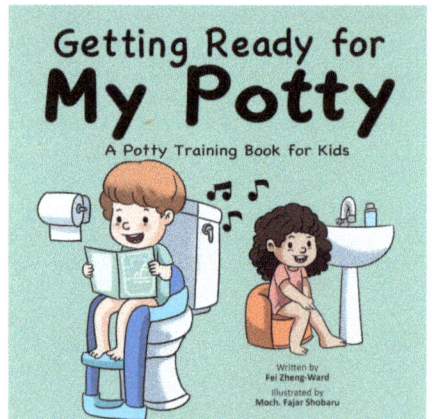
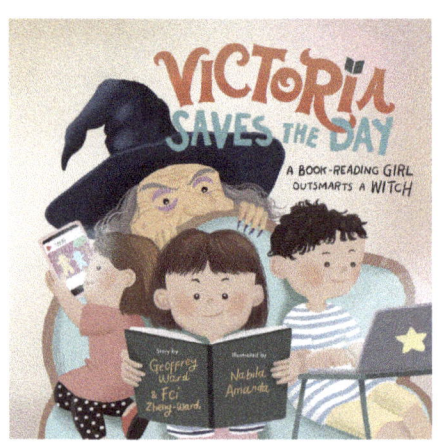
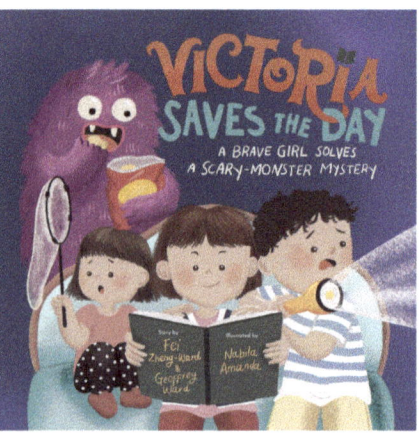
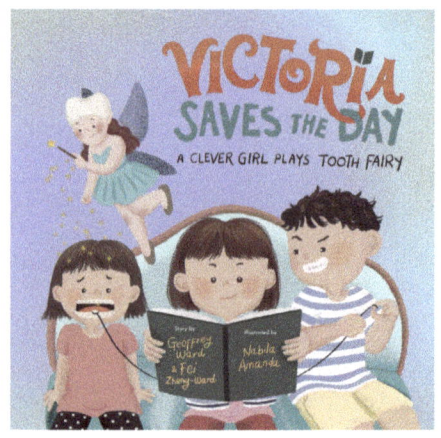

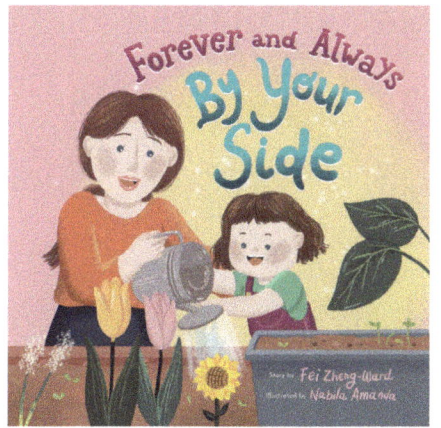
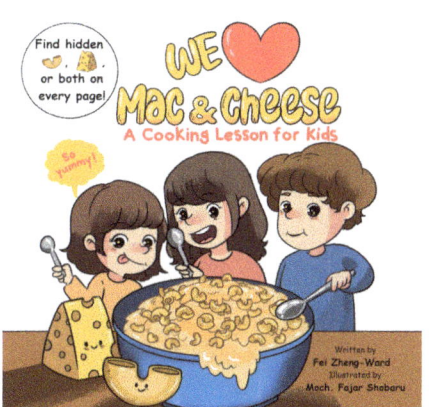
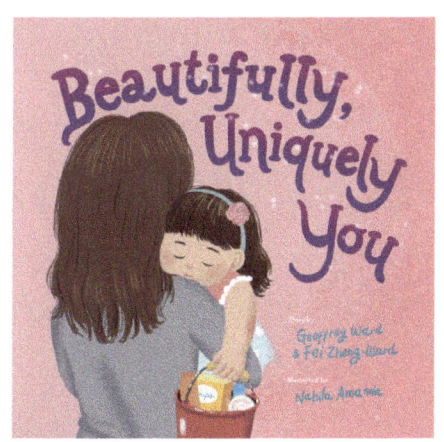
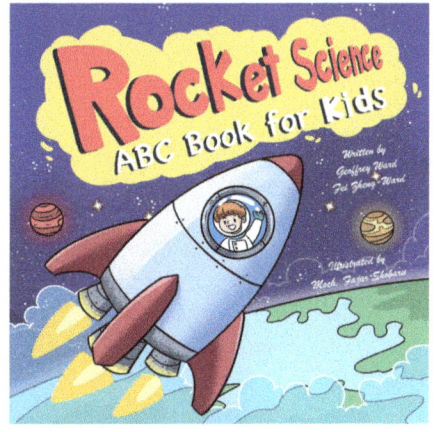
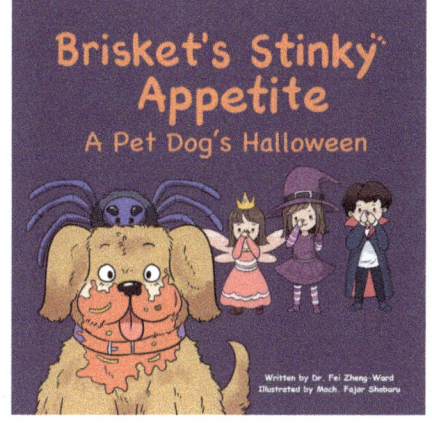
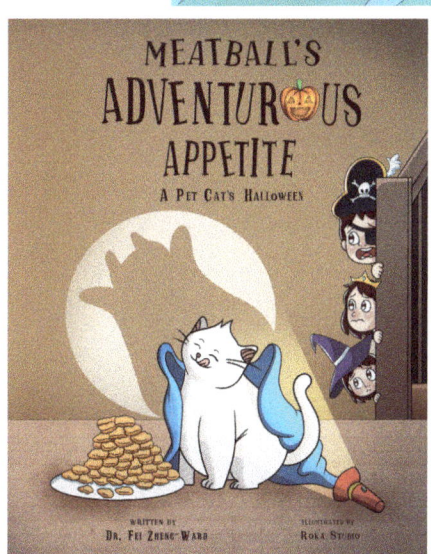
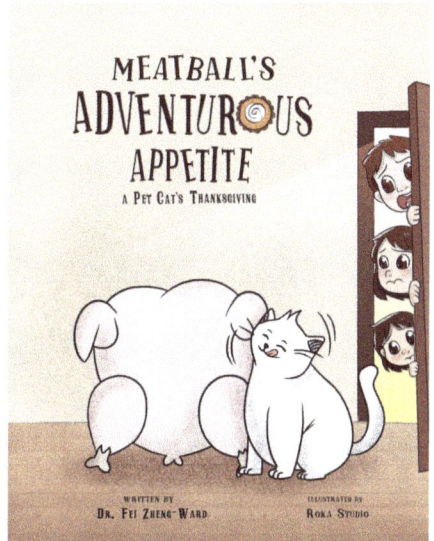
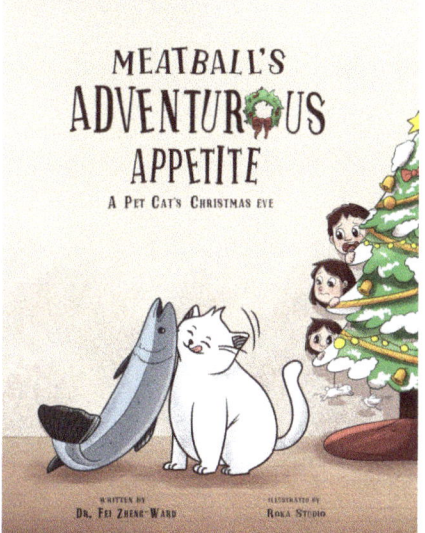

Coming soon:

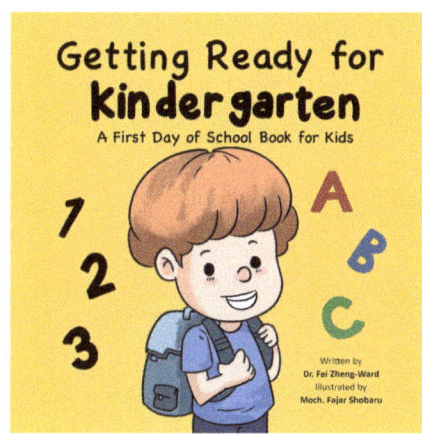

www.ingramcontent.com/pod-product-compliance
Lightning Source LLC
Chambersburg PA
CBHW042359030426
42337CB00032B/5158